Musculoskeletal PET Imaging

Guest Editor

ROLAND HUSTINX, MD, PhD

PET CLINICS

www.pet.theclinics.com

Consulting Editor
ABASS ALAVI, MD,
MD (Hon), PhD (Hon), DSc (Hon)

July 2010 • Volume 5 • Number 3

SAUNDERS an imprint of ELSEVIER, Inc.

W.B. SAUNDERS COMPANY
A Division of Elsevier Inc.

1600 John F. Kennedy Boulevard • Suite 1800 • Philadelphia, Pennsylvania 19103-2899

http://www.theclinics.com

PET CLINICS Volume 5, Number 3
July 2010 ISSN 1556-8598, ISBN-13: 978-1-4377-2592-6

Editor: Barton Dudlick

PET Clinics (ISSN 1556-8598) is published quarterly by Elsevier Inc., 360 Park Avenue South, New York, NY 10010-1710. Months of issue are January, April, July, and October. Periodicals postage paid at New York, NY, and additional mailing offices. Subscription prices per year are $196.00 (US individuals), $279.00 (US institutions), $97.00 (US students), $223.00 (Canadian individuals), $312.00 (Canadian institutions), $118.00 (Canadian students), $237.00 (foreign individuals), $312.00 (foreign institutions), and $118.00 (foreign students). To receive student and resident rate, orders must be accompanied by name of affiliated institution, date of term, and the signature of program/residency coordinator on institution letterhead. Orders will be billed at individual rate until proof of status is received. Foreign air speed delivery is included in all Clinics subscription prices. All prices are subject to change without notice. POSTMASTER: Send address changes to PET Clinics, Elsevier Health Sciences Division, Subscription Customer Service, 3251 Riverport Lane, Maryland Heights, MO 63043. **Customer Service: 1-800-654-2452 (U.S. and Canada); 314-447-8871 (outside U.S. and Canada). Fax: 314-447-8029. E-mail: journalscustomerservice-usa@elsevier.com (for print support); journalsonlinesupport-usa@elsevier.com (for online support).**

Reprints. For copies of 100 or more of articles in this publication, please contact the Commercial Reprints Department, Elsevier Inc., 360 Park Avenue South, New York, NY 10010-1710. Tel.: 212-633-3812; Fax: 212-462-1935; E-mail: reprints@elsevier.com.

Contributors

CONSULTING EDITOR

ABASS ALAVI, MD, MD (Hon), PhD (Hon), DSc (Hon)
Director of Research Education, Nuclear Medicine Section, Department of Radiology, Hospital of the University of Pennsylvania, Philadelphia, Pennsylvania

GUEST EDITOR

ROLAND HUSTINX, MD, PhD
Division of Nuclear Medicine, University Hospital of Liège, Liège, Belgium

AUTHORS

AKRAM AL-IBRAHEEM, MD, FEBNM
Department of Nuclear Medicine, King Hussein Medical Center, Amman, Jordan

IVAYLA APOSTOLOVA, MD
Department of Nuclear Medicine, Charité-Universitätsmedizin Berlin, Berlin, Germany

AMBROS J. BEER, MD
Department of Nuclear Medicine, Technische Universität München, Munich, Germany

GLEN M. BLAKE, PhD
Senior Lecturer in Imaging Sciences, Osteoporosis Unit, King's College London, Guy's Campus, Great Maze Pond, London, United Kingdom

WINFRIED BRENNER, MD, PhD
Head, Department of Nuclear Medicine, Charité-Universitätsmedizin Berlin, Berlin, Germany

ANDREAS K. BUCK, MD
Department of Nuclear Medicine, Technische Universität München, Munich, Germany

GANG CHENG, MD, PhD
Department of Radiology, Children's Hospital of Philadelphia, Philadelphia, Pennsylvania

HUBERT H. CHUANG, MD, PhD
Assistant Professor of Nuclear Medicine, Division of Diagnostic Imaging, Department of Nuclear Medicine, The University of Texas MD Anderson Cancer Center, Houston, Texas

J. COLLIGNON, MD
Division of Medical Oncology, CHU Sart Tilman Liège, Liège, Belgium

COLLEEN M. COSTELLOE, MD
Assistant Professor of Radiology, Division of Diagnostic Imaging, Department of Diagnostic Radiology, The University of Texas MD Anderson Cancer Center, Houston, Texas

GARY J.R. COOK, MSc, MD, FRCR, FRCP
Department of Nuclear Medicine and PET, The Royal Marsden NHS Foundation Trust, Sutton, United Kingdom

LAURA A. DRUBACH, MD
Staff Physician, Division of Nuclear Medicine, Children's Hospital Boston; Assistant Professor in Radiology, Joint Program in Nuclear Medicine, Harvard Medical School, Boston, Massachusetts

STEFANO FANTI, MD
Department of Nuclear Medicine, Azienda Ospedaliero-Universitaria di Bologna Policlinico S.Orsola-Malpighi, Bologna, Italy

IGNAC FOGELMAN, MD
Professor, Department of Nuclear Medicine, King's College London, Guy's Campus, Great Maze Pond, London, United Kingdom

PACÔME FOSSE, MD
Division of Nuclear Medicine, University Hospital of Liège, Liège, Belgium

MICHELLE L. FROST, PhD
Senior Lecturer in Osteoporosis, Osteoporosis Unit, King's College London, Guy's Campus, Great Maze Pond, London

C. GENNIGENS, MD
Division of Medical Oncology, CHU Sart Tilman Liège, Liège, Belgium

FREDERICK D. GRANT, MD
Staff Physician, Division of Nuclear Medicine, Children's Hospital Boston; Instructor in Radiology and Associate Training Program Director, Joint Program in Nuclear Medicine, Harvard Medical School, Boston, Massachusetts

KEN HERRMANN, MD
Department of Nuclear Medicine, Technische Universität München, Munich, Germany

ROLAND HUSTINX, MD, PhD
Division of Nuclear Medicine, University Hospital of Liège, Liège, Belgium

ANDREI IAGARU, MD
Clinical Instructor, Division of Nuclear Medicine, Department of Radiology, Stanford Hospital and Clinics, Stanford, California

G. JERUSALEM, MD, PhD
Division of Medical Oncology, CHU Sart Tilman Liège; University of Liège, Liège, Belgium

KAZUHIRO KATAHIRA, MD, PhD
Department of Radiology, Kumamoto Central Hospital, Kumamoto, Japan

THOMAS C. KWEE, MD
Department of Radiology, University Medical Center Utrecht, Utrecht, The Netherlands

JOHN E. MADEWELL, MD
Professor of Radiology, Division of Diagnostic Imaging, Department of Diagnostic Radiology, The University of Texas MD Anderson Cancer Center, Houston, Texas

ERIK MITTRA, MD, PhD
Clinical Instructor, Division of Nuclear Medicine, Department of Radiology, Stanford Hospital and Clinics, Stanford, California

KATSUYUKI NAKANISHI, MD, PhD
Department of Radiology, Osaka Medical Center for Cancer and Cardiovascular Diseases, Osaka, Japan

CRISTINA NANNI, MD
Department of Nuclear Medicine, Azienda Ospedaliero-Universitaria di Bologna Policlinico S. Orsola-Malpighi, Bologna, Italy

TARO TAKAHARA, MD, PhD
Department of Radiology, University Medical Center Utrecht, Utrecht, The Netherlands

S. TED TREVES, MD
Division of Nuclear Medicine, Children's Hospital Boston; Professor in Radiology and Director, Joint Program in Nuclear Medicine, Harvard Medical School, Boston, Massachusetts

HONGMING ZHUANG, MD, PhD
Department of Radiology, Children's Hospital of Philadelphia, Philadelphia, Pennsylvania

Contents

In recent years the more widespread availability of PET systems and the development of hybrid PET/computed tomography (CT) imaging, allowing improved morphologic characterization of sites with increased tracer uptake, have improved the accuracy of diagnosis and strengthened the role of 18F-fluoride PET for quantitative assessment of bone pathology. This article reviews the role of 18F-fluoride PET in the skeleton, with a focus on (1) the underlying physiologic and pathophysiological processes of different conditions of bone metabolism and (2) methodological aspects of quantitative measurement of 18F-fluoride kinetics. Recent comparative studies have demonstrated that 18F-fluoride PET and, to an even greater extent, PET/CT are more accurate than 99mTc-bisphosphonate single-photon emission CT for the identification of malignant and benign lesions of the skeleton. Quantitative 18F-flouride PET has been shown valuable for direct non-invasive assessment of bone metabolism and monitoring response to therapy.

An assessment of bone turnover at specific sites of the skeleton would allow a better understanding of the pathophysiology of osteoporosis and the direct effects of drugs on bone turnover at common osteoporotic fracture sites. ^{18}F-Fluoride PET provides a noninvasive method for the assessment of regional bone perfusion and turnover, and offers important advantages over conventional techniques. ^{18}F-Fluoride PET has been used to examine bone turnover in patients with osteoporosis and other metabolic bone disorders, to compare bone perfusion and turnover between skeletal sites, to assess novel therapies being developed for the treatment of osteoporosis, and to examine the fracture healing process. ^{18}F-Fluoride PET may also have a role in diagnosis of bone turnover abnormalities in patients with renal osteodystrophy. ^{18}F-Fluoride PET now has an established role as a research technique, and there is clearly a need for further studies to fully examine its potential role in the assessment of the pathophysiology of osteoporosis and the evaluation of novel pharmaceutical treatments for this and other metabolic bone disorders.

[18]F-fluoride is a bone-specific PET tracer that was first described 40 years ago, but it has been more extensively investigated in the setting of bone metastases only in more recent years. ^{18}F-fluoride PET is a highly sensitive method for detecting bone metastases in many cancers, and the use of ^{18}F-fluoride with hybrid PET/computed tomography (CT) further improves specificity with the additional morphologic information available from the CT component. ^{18}F-fluoride provides complementary information to tumor-specific PET tracers, and it is likely that this imaging method will continue to be used more routinely and for newer applications to grow.

A literature review was performed of studies reporting sensitivity and specificity of [18F]fluorodeoxyglucose (FDG) PET from January 1, 2000 to January 1, 2010. PET was found to have higher sensitivity for the detection of osseous metastases when compared to CT, skeletal scintigraphy, whole body MRI and combined conventional imaging modalities. A potential exception is when comparing PET with bone scan in the setting of blastic metastases. PET may be a better indicator of active bony metastases. The efficacy of PET can be increased with fused anatomic imaging.

The bone marrow is a common site for metastasis in cancer. Accurate detection of bone marrow metastases is of major importance because of its therapeutic and prognostic implications. MRI allows direct visualization of all bone marrow components at a good spatial resolution. Furthermore, thanks to technologic advances, it is now possible to perform MRI of the entire body. For these reasons, it is a potentially valuable technique for the detection of bone marrow metastases. This article reviews whole-body MRI techniques and the diagnostic performance of whole-body MRI compared with PET for the detection of bone marrow metastases.

Bone is one of the most common sites of metastases from cancer. Most anticancer treatments are highly toxic but only a fraction of all patients respond to them. Guidelines are needed to evaluate the response in the routine practice of oncology as well as in clinical trials in which new treatment options are evaluated. All current imaging procedures have major limitations. This article reviews old and new criteria for response evaluation. The major problem of accurate response evaluation in bone disease is discussed in detail. Some examples from our daily practice illustrate the difficulties. The indications for bone biopsy are also reviewed.

Imaging is critical for the proper evaluation of patients with primary tumors of bone. There is a growing role for ^{18}F-fluorodeoxyglucose PET and PET/computed tomography (CT) in the grading, staging, prognostication, evaluation of therapeutic response, and detection of recurrent disease in bone. These modalities can also be used to help differentiate benign from malignant disorders of bone.

Sarcomas are a heterogeneous group of tumors that generally present a poor prognosis. Recently, ^{18}F fluorodeoxyglucose (FDG–Positron emission tomography (PET)/computed tomography (CT) was introduced in clinical practice as a possible tool to improve the accuracy of staging these malignant diseases, assess the response to therapy, and as a new prognostic factor. Despite promising results presented in the recent literature, the role of PET imaging is not yet defined in the diagnostic flow chart of sarcomas. This article will describe the results reported in the literature on the use of FDG-PET/CT for the evaluation of patients with sarcoma. A short description of other PET tracers is also added.

^{18}F-Fluorodeoxy-glucose PET and PET/CT in Pediatric Musculoskeletal Malignancies   349

Frederick D. Grant, Laura A. Drubach, and S. Ted Treves

Although uncommon, musculoskeletal malignancies are major contributors to morbidity and mortality in children and young adults. ^{18}F-Fluorodeoxyglucose (FDG)-PET can play an important role in disease management, including staging, assessing response to therapy, and evaluating for recurrence. Advantages of ^{18}F-FDG-PET and ^{18}F-FDG-PET/computed tomography (CT) include the capability to assess tumor activity and a large field of view that can include the whole body or torso. ^{18}F-FDG-PET does not always discriminate benign and malignant musculoskeletal lesion, but it can serve to guide diagnostic procedures, such as needle biopsy. In patients with osteosarcoma, FDG-PET/CT cannot replace a 99mTc-methyldiphosphonate bone scan for localization of skeletal metastases. FDG-PET may be useful for the evaluation of non-rhabdomyosarcoma sarcomas on a case-by-case basis. ^{18}F-FDG-PET or PET/CT is most useful for identifying sites of distant disease in patients with newly diagnosed or recurrent Ewing sarcoma, rhabdomyosarcoma, or osseous lymphoma.

Alternative PET Tracers in Musculoskeletal Disease   363

Akram Al-Ibraheem, Andreas K. Buck, Ambros J. Beer, and Ken Herrmann

Noninvasive detection, identification, and evaluation of malignant musculoskeletal tumors is difficult because of the varied grades of tumor malignancies. Positron emission tomography (PET) using radiolabeled tracers for musculoskeletal tumor detection has gained popularity because of the more detailed information it provides on tumor aggressiveness and biologic response to therapy compared with conventional techniques. Radiolabeled fluorine, amino acids, and choline have also proved to be successful in differentiating benign lesions from malignant tumors using PET. The sensitivity and specificity of the radiolabeled tracers may help in early detection and treatment of tumors in patients with cancer. In this article, the potential role of these alternative PET tracers in musculoskeletal disorders is reviewed with emphasis on oncologic applications.

Applications of PET and PET/CT in the Evaluation of Infection and Inflammation in the Skeletal System   375

Gang Cheng, Pacôme Fosse, Hongming Zhuang, and Roland Hustinx

Unlike anatomic imaging modalities, which mainly detect structural changes, positron emission tomography (PET) is a molecular imaging technique able to detect the disease in an early stage and long before anatomic changes are visible. It is well known that fluorodeoxyglucose (FDG) accumulates at the sites of various inflammatory and infectious processes. FDG-PET or FDG-PET/computed tomography (CT) has been successfully used in the evaluation of various nonosseous soft tissue infections. Its application in the evaluation of osseous infection is also promising. This review discusses the potential roles of PET or PET/CT in the evaluation of infection and inflammation in the skeletal system.

PET Clinics

THE CLINICS ARE NOW AVAILABLE ONLINE!

Access your subscription at:
www.theclinics.com

GOAL STATEMENT

The goal of the *PET Clinics* is to keep practicing radiologists and radiology residents up to date with current clinical practice in positron emission tomography by providing timely articles reviewing the state of the art in patient care.

ACCREDITATION

PET Clinics is planned and implemented in accordance with the Essential Areas and Policies of the Accreditation Council for Continuing Medical Education (ACCME) through the joint sponsorship of the University of Virginia School of Medicine and Elsevier. The University of Virginia School of Medicine is accredited by the ACCME to provide continuing medical education for physicians.

The University of Virginia School of Medicine designates this educational activity for a maximum of 15 *AMA PRA Category 1 Credits*™ for each issue, 60 credits per year. Physicians should only claim credit commensurate with the extent of their participation in the activity.

The American Medical Association has determined that physicians not licensed in the US who participate in this CME activity are eligible for a maximum of 15 *AMA PRA Category 1 Credits*™ for each issue, 60 credits per year.

Category 1 credit can be earned by reading the text material, taking the CME examination online at http://www.theclinics.com/home/cme, and completing the evaluation. After taking the test, you will be required to review any and all incorrect answers. Following completion of the test and evaluation, your credit will be awarded and you may print your certificate.

FACULTY DISCLOSURE/CONFLICT OF INTEREST

The University of Virginia School of Medicine, as an ACCME accredited provider, endorses and strives to comply with the Accreditation Council for Continuing Medical Education (ACCME) Standards of Commercial Support, Commonwealth of Virginia statutes, University of Virginia policies and procedures, and associated federal and private regulations and guidelines on the need for disclosure and monitoring of proprietary and financial interests that may affect the scientific integrity and balance of content delivered in continuing medical education activities under our auspices.

The University of Virginia School of Medicine requires that all CME activities accredited through this institution be developed independently and be scientifically rigorous, balanced and objective in the presentation/discussion of its content, theories and practices.

All authors/editors participating in an accredited CME activity are expected to disclose to the readers relevant financial relationships with commercial entities occurring within the past 12 months (such as grants or research support, employee, consultant, stock holder, member of speakers bureau, etc.). The University of Virginia School of Medicine will employ appropriate mechanisms to resolve potential conflicts of interest to maintain the standards of fair and balanced education to the reader. Questions about specific strategies can be directed to the Office of Continuing Medical Education, University of Virginia School of Medicine, Charlottesville, Virginia.

The faculty and staff of the University of Virginia Office of Continuing Medical Education have no financial affiliations to disclose.

The authors/editors listed below have identified no professional or financial affiliations for themselves or their spouse/partner:

Abass Alavi, MD (Consulting Editor); Akram Al-Ibraheem, MD, FEBNM; Ivayla Apostolova, MD; Ambros J. Beer, MD; Glen M. Blake, PhD; Winfried Brenner, MD, PhD; Andreas K. Buck, MD; Gang Cheng, MD, PhD; Hubert H. Chuang, MD, PhD; J. Collignon, MD; Colleen M. Costelloe, MD; Laura A. Drubach, MD; Barton Dudlick (Acquisitions Editor); Stefano Fanti, MD; Ignac Fogelman, MD; Pacôme Fosse, MD; Michelle L. Frost, PhD; C. Gennigens, MD; Ken Herrmann, MD; Roland Hustinx, MD, PhD (Guest Editor); Andrei Iagaru, MD; G. Jerusalem, MD, PhD; Kazuhiro Katahira, MD, PhD; Thomas C. Kwee, MD; John E. Madewell, MD; Erik Mittra, MD, PhD; Katsuyuki Nakanishi, MD, PhD; Cristina Nanni, MD; Patrice Rehm, MD (Test Author); Taro Takahara, MD, PhD; S.Ted Treves, MD; and Hongming Zhuang, MD, PhD.

The authors/editors listed below identified the following professional or financial affiliations for themselves or their spouse/partner:

Gary J. R. Cook, MSc, MD, FRCR, FRCP is on the Advisory Committee/Board and is a stockholder for Medical Imaging Group Ltd.
Frederick D. Grant, MD is an industry funded research/investigator for GE Medical Imaging.

Disclosure of Discussion of Non-FDA Approved Uses for Pharmaceutical Products and/or Medical Devices.

The University of Virginia School of Medicine, as an ACCME provider, requires that all faculty presenters identify and disclose any off-label uses for pharmaceutical and medical device products. The University of Virginia School of Medicine recommends that each physician fully review all the available data on new products or procedures prior to clinical use.

TO ENROLL

To enroll in the PET Clinics Continuing Medical Education program, call customer service at 1-800-654-2452 or visit us online at www.theclinics.com/home/cme. The CME program is available to subscribers for an additional fee of $196.00.

Preface

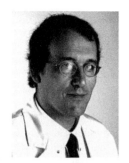

Roland Hustinx, MD, PhD
Guest Edtior

Musculoskeletal disorders have always been a major field for applications of nuclear medicine. Initial reports on the use of radio-isotopes to investigate bone metabolism or malignant bone involvement were published more than half a century ago.[1,2] At the present time, bone scanning with ^{99m}Tc-labeled diphosphonates remains among the most commonly performed nuclear medicine procedures worldwide. Recent developments have set the table for further widening the scope of metabolic imaging in this setting.

[18]F-NaF was introduced in 1962 but was promptly replaced by single-photon emitters better suited to the detectors available at that time. Nowadays, however, most positron emission tomographic/computed tomographic (PET/CT) systems provide a fully tomographic, high-resolution survey of the entire body, from head to toes, in 20 minutes or even less. PET/CT with ^{18}F-NaF now provides, in a time frame that compares favorably to the most modern single-photon emission computed tomographic (SPECT)/CT systems, a wealth of information that can be used in both oncologic and benign disorders. Furthermore, thanks to the quantitative aspects of PET, unique insights into bone metabolism are revealed, which may prove particularly useful and clinically relevant in the assessment of osteoporosis.[3] For detecting bone metastases, PET/CT with ^{18}F-NaF or fluorodeoxyglucose (FDG) is the most accurate nuclear medicine technique, and exciting studies are underway to evaluate its role, in particular, compared to the most recent developments in whole-body magnetic resonance imaging.[4] Recurrent shortages in Molybdenum and increased costs for the once ubiquitous ^{99m}Tc lead to questioning and re-assessing the axiom according to which PET cannot compete with bone scintigraphy in terms of cost effectiveness. At this point, very little data are available directly comparing performances of SPECT/CT and PET/CT. Similarly, although FDG remains the tracer of choice for investigating bone and soft-tissue sarcomas, alternative tracers offer intriguing possibilities. In particular, efforts are being made to assess angiogenesis with radio-labeled ligands to the $\alpha v \beta 3$ integrin, and such biological targets for molecular imaging may prove extremely useful in the near future.[5] On the other hand, the lack of specificity of FDG for tumors may be turned into profit in infectious and inflammatory disorders such as chronic osteomyelitis and rheumatoid arthritis.[6,7] Again, the improved spatial resolution and increased speed of modern PET/CT scanners make it possible to envision a routine clinical role, although further investigation is needed.

Clearly, imaging of the musculoskeletal system is rapidly and profoundly evolving. Many techniques are available or under investigation, from SPECT/CT to PET/CT, with a wide variety of radiotracers, and from planar radiography to whole-body diffusion-weighted magnetic resonance imaging. Nevertheless clinical diagnostic algorithms remain largely unchanged, especially in oncology, as clinicians may find it difficult to sort out among this profusion of techniques. The major task ahead will therefore be to define the exact role for each technique, taking into account not only the diagnostic performances but the practical

PET Clin 5 (2010) xi–xii
doi:10.1016/j.cpet.2010.06.001

and economic aspects. Considering the major advances observed during the past 5 years, exciting developments are to be expected.

Roland Hustinx, MD, PhD
Service de Médecine Nucléaire
Centre Hospitalier Universitaire de Liège
Sart Tilman B35, Liège 4000, Belgium

E-mail address:
rhustinx@chu.ulg.ac.be

REFERENCES

1. Bohr H, Halborg Sorensen A. Study of fracture healing by means of radioactive tracers. J Bone Joint Surg Am 1950;32-A(3):567–74.
2. Mulry WC, Dudley HC. Studies of radiogallium as a diagnostic agent in bone tumors. J Lab Clin Med 1951;37(2):239–52.
3. Frost ML, Cook GJ, Blake GM, et al. The relationship between regional bone turnover measured using 18F-fluoride positron emission tomography and changes in BMD is equivalent to that seen for biochemical markers of bone turnover. J Clin Densitom 2007; 10(1):46–54.
4. Heusner TA, Kuemmel S, Koeninger A, et al. Diagnostic value of diffusion-weighted magnetic resonance imaging (DWI) compared to FDG PET/CT for whole-body breast cancer staging. Eur J Nucl Med Mol Imaging 2010;37(6):1077–86.
5. Beer AJ, Haubner R, Sarbia M, et al. Positron emission tomography using [18F]Galacto-RGD identifies the level of integrin alpha(v)beta3 expression in man. Clin Cancer Res 2006;12(13): 3942–9.
6. Hartmann A, Eid K, Dora C, et al. Diagnostic value of 18F-FDG PET/CT in trauma patients with suspected chronic osteomyelitis. Eur J Nucl Med Mol Imaging 2007;34(5):704–14.
7. Beckers C, Ribbens C, André B, et al. Assessment of disease activity in rheumatoid arthritis with (18)F-FDG PET. J Nucl Med 2004;45(6):956–64.

Measuring Bone Metabolism with Fluoride PET: Methodological Considerations

Ivayla Apostolova, MD, Winfried Brenner, MD, PhD*

KEYWORDS

- Fluoride PET • Bone metabolism • Quantitation
- Nonlinear regression analysis • Patlak analysis
- Standardized uptake value

The positron emitter ^{18}F-fluoride has a long history as a tracer for bone imaging. ^{18}F-Fluoride was first introduced by Blau and colleagues[1] in 1962 as an agent for skeletal scintigraphy, decades before the introduction of modern PET systems. Because of its favorable pharmacokinetic properties, ^{18}F-fluoride had become the standard agent for bone scanning until the development of ^{99m}Tc-labeled bisphosphonates in the 1970s.[2,3] The establishment of ^{99m}Tc-labeled bisphosphonates as standard bone imaging tracers did not reflect pharmacokinetic limitations of ^{18}F-labeled NaF, but was the result of first, the technical limitations associated with imaging the 511-keV photons from positron annihilation on a system optimized for the 140-keV photons of ^{99m}Tc, and second, the cost of cyclotron-based production together with logistic challenges in the delivery of a radioisotope with a physical half-life of 110 minutes.

In recent years, due to the more widespread availability of PET systems, the technical limitations for imaging with ^{18}F-fluoride have for the most part been overcome and ^{18}F-labeled NaF has strengthened its role as a widely used radiotracer, especially for quantitative assessment of bone pathology.[4] ^{18}F-fluoride combines the properties of high and rapid bone uptake as well as rapid blood clearance, which contribute to the high bone-to-background ratio images obtained within an hour after tracer administration. Moreover, current PET scanners have higher spatial resolution and substantially greater sensitivity than conventional gamma cameras, and also enable quantitative assessment of bone metabolism using dynamic acquisition, which has aroused anew the interest in the tracer as a valuable bone imaging agent.[5,6] The recent development of hybrid imaging PET/computed tomography (CT) systems, allowing CT-based attenuation correction and morphologic characterization of sites with increased tracer uptake, has improved the accuracy of diagnosis and the role of ^{18}F-fluoride in bone imaging.

RADIOPHARMACEUTICS

[18]F-Fluoride is a career-free cyclotron product synthesized in a one-step reaction by irradiation of [18]O with cyclotron-accelerated protons. Subsequently, the fluoride containing ^{18}O-water should pass through an anion exchange resin column. Fluoride is released by elution with a sodium chloride solution (0.9%) followed by sterile filtration. Using an aliquot, quality control should be performed in analogy to ^{18}F-fluorodeoxyglucose (FDG). pH value, osmolarity, solvent content,

The authors have no conflicts of interest to disclose.
Department of Nuclear Medicine, Charité-Universitätsmedizin Berlin, Charitéplatz 1, 10117 Berlin, Germany
* Corresponding author.
E-mail address: winfried.brenner@charite.de

PET Clin 5 (2010) 247–257
doi:10.1016/j.cpet.2010.02.008

presence of endotoxins, chemical and radiochemical purity (high-performance liquid chromatography [HPLC], thin-layer chromatography), and half-life should be documented. The solution should not contain short-lived isotopes like ^{13}N or any long-life isotopes. If the concentration of long-life isotopes exceeds a certain amount, an HPLC cleaning procedure of the sodium fluoride solution is recommended. Sterility of the solution should be preserved. After successful quality control, the solution is ready for use without further chemical processing.

^{18}F-FLUORIDE METABOLISM

Bone remodeling is achieved through the activity of osteoclasts and osteoblasts, which resorb old bone tissue and lay down new bone. In skeletal diseases both the rate of remodeling and the balance between bone resorption and bone formation might be altered. Radionuclide tracers such as ^{18}F-fluoride ions and ^{99m}Tc-bisphosphonates provide a technique for studying bone turnover.[2,7] ^{18}F-Fluoride ion is extracted by the skeletal system in proportion to bone blood flow and osteoblastic activity. Fluoride bone uptake mechanisms are similar to those of ^{99m}Tc-bisphosphonates, reflecting the increased regional blood flow and bone turnover.[4] In the plasma, ^{18}F-fluoride ions bind only minimally to plasma proteins and clear from circulation in a biexponential manner, faster than ^{99m}Tc-bisphosphonates. It has been reported that exponent (i), which represents bone uptake, has a plasma clearance half-time of 24 minutes and exponent (ii), representing mainly renal clearance, has a blood clearance half-time of 198 minutes for ^{18}F-fluoride.[8] It has been mostly assumed that the initial uptake of ^{18}F-fluoride by bone depends solely on its rate of delivery to bone, that is, on the blood supply, and that the efficiency of extraction of the isotope by bone is very high (ca 100%) at each blood passage.[9] However, it has been shown already by Costeas and colleagues[10] in 1970 that the retention of the tracer in the bone is a 2-phase process. In the first phase, fluoride ions diffuse through capillary walls into bone extracellular fluid and are chemisorbed onto bone surface by exchanging with hydroxyl (OH) groups in hydroxyapatite ($Ca_{10}(PO_4)_6(OH)_2$) crystals of bone to form fluoroapatite. In the second phase, the ^{18}F-fluoride ion migrates into the crystalline matrix of bone, where it is retained until the bone is remodeled. Immediately after ^{18}F-fluoride exchanges with stable fluoride or other anions on crystal surfaces, the isotope begins to be incorporated into new crystals of bone salt and to diffuse into deeper layers of

bone, but these processes are so slow that they do not play a significant role quantitatively during the first few hours. The upper limit of the total amount of isotope that can be deposited in bone in a given time is imposed by perfusion of the bone (perfusion-limited uptake). As soon as the specific activity in the blood has fallen below that on the bone surface, the concentration on the bone begins to decrease owing to reverse exchange. Within this limit, the amount of tracer that is actually accumulated in the bone is determined by the size of the exchangeable pool.[10] This, on the other hand, depends on the size of the metabolically active surfaces in the bone, which is the parameter of clinical interest. The concentration of ^{18}F-fluoride in bone was found to reach a maximum 2 to 3 hours after injection and then began to decrease slowly. One hour after administration of ^{18}F-labeled NaF, only about 10% of the injected activity remains in the blood.[1]

Approximately 30% of ^{18}F-fluoride is transported by erythrocytes; however, this fraction is also easily available for clearance in the bones, because equilibration between erythrocytes and plasma is much faster than the capillary transit time.[11] Tosteson[12] showed that anions were rapidly transported across the red cell membrane with a rate constant of 0.3 per second for fluoride. A significant advantage of ^{18}F-fluoride compared with ^{99m}Tc-bisphosphonate bone agents is that the latter show significant binding to plasma proteins, in contrast to ^{18}F-fluoride. Approximately 30% of ^{99m}Tc-bisphosphonates are protein bound immediately after injection; this fraction increases to approximately 70% by 24 h after injection.[13,14] The nonprotein-bound fraction of ^{99m}Tc–methylene diphosphonate (^{99m}Tc-MDP) is rapidly cleared from the blood with a half-life similar to that of ^{18}F-fluoride, but the protein-bound fraction is cleared much more slowly, because of the slow exchange between protein-bound and free fraction in plasma.[15] Therefore it is necessary to wait 3 to 4 hours after injection of ^{99m}Tc-MDP before imaging. By comparison, imaging can be performed less than 1 hour after intravenous injection of ^{18}F-fluoride.

CLINICAL ROLE OF STATIC ^{18}F-FLUORIDE PET

A well-studied indication for static ^{18}F-fluoride PET imaging is the detection of bone involvement in primary bone tumors or in secondary metastatic bone disease (**Fig. 1**). Due to the faster blood clearance and higher capillary permeability, fluoride uptake in bone metastases is significantly higher, with a 5 to 10 times higher transport rate constant for trapping of the tracer in the metastatic

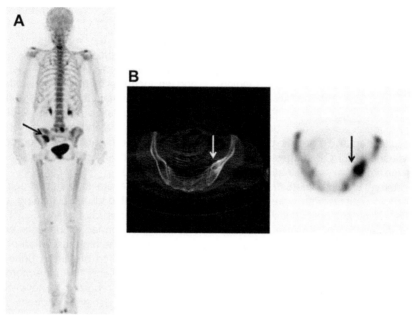

Fig. 1. (*A*) Whole-body ^{18}F-fluoride PET in a patient with prostate cancer and multiple bone metastases. (*B*) PET/CT shows a sclerotic lesion in the left pelvic bone with significant ^{18}F-fluoride uptake (*arrow*). (*Courtesy of* UKE Hamburg.)

lesions compared with that of normal bone.[16] Increased fluoride uptake has been reported in both sclerotic and lytic metastases[16] and, similar to ^{99m}Tc-MDP, is also seen in benign bone diseases and nonmalignant orthopedic problems. ^{18}F-Fluoride is therefore not considered a tumor-specific tracer.

In a recent study, Schirrmeister and colleagues[17] showed that ^{18}F-fluoride PET was more sensitive than bone scintigraphy in detecting osseous lesions and that the detection rates for osteoblastic and osteolytic metastases were similar. In this prospective trial including 44 patients with different malignancies, ^{18}F-fluoride PET showed 96 metastases whereas bone scintigraphy revealed 46 metastases, all of them also detected with ^{18}F-fluoride PET. Compared with ^{18}F-fluoride PET and the reference methods of magnetic resonance imaging (MRI), CT, and conventional radiography, bone scanning had a sensitivity of 83% in detecting malignant and benign osseous lesions in the skull, thorax, and extremities, and a sensitivity of 40% in the spine and pelvis.[17] In another large prospective trial including a total of 103 patients with lung cancer examined with planar bone scintigraphy (BS), single-photon emission CT (SPECT) of the vertebral column, and PET using [18]F- fluoride, Schirrmeister and colleagues[18] showed that the area under the receiver-operating characteristic curve was 0.771 for BS, 0.875 for SPECT, and 0.989

for ^{18}F-fluoride PET (*P*<.05), confirming the greater sensitivity of ^{18}F-fluoride PET and its potential to change the clinical patient management. As a result of SPECT and ^{18}F-fluoride PET imaging, clinical management was changed in 7.8% and 9.7% of the patients, respectively.

The same group reported in another study evaluating the frequency, distribution, and appearance of benign lesions in ^{18}F-fluoride PET scans that most of the degenerative lesions (84%) could be detected with ^{18}F-fluoride PET, whereas bone scans revealed approximately 30% fewer lesions.[19] Schirrmeister and colleagues[20] reported in 1998 that even very small details in the spine such as spinous and transverse processes were clearly visible in ^{18}F-fluoride PET scans of the normal skeletal system, whereas only half of the structures could be visualized in bone scans. However, because of its high sensitivity, ^{18}F-fluoride PET performed for assessment of malignant bone involvement was prone to a high rate of false-positive interpretations by detecting nonmalignant lesions, including lesions that are usually not detectable with ^{99m}Tc-bisphosphonate BS. Newer studies showed that the use of hybrid PET/CT has significantly improved the limited specificity of ^{18}F-fluoride PET because the morphologic CT appearance of the metabolic lesions achieved a more accurate differentiation between benign involvement and metastases. In several studies, Even-Sapir and coworkers investigated the value of combined PET/CT imaging compared with PET alone. In a study of 44 unselected cancer patients they showed that the specificity of PET/CT was higher compared with PET alone (97% vs 72%, $P<.001$) with the sensitivity of PET ranging between 72% and 90%, and a sensitivity of 99% for PET/CT. Moreover, among 12 patients referred for ^{18}F-fluoride assessment because of bone pain despite negative findings on ^{99m}Tc-MDP BS, ^{18}F-fluoride PET/CT suggested malignant bone involvement in all 4 patients with subsequent proven skeletal metastases.[21] In another study of 44 patients with high-risk prostate cancer, Even-Sapir and colleagues[22] showed that the sensitivity, specificity, positive predictive value, and negative predictive value of planar bone scan were 70%, 57%, 64%, and 55%, respectively, of multi-field-of-view SPECT were 92%, 82%, 86%, and 90%, of ^{18}F-fluoride PET were 100%, 62%, 74%, and 100%, and of ^{18}F-fluoride PET/CT were 100% for all parameters.

Although ^{18}F-fluoride provides a more sensitive "conventional" bone scan and is superior in FDG nonavid bony lesions, FDG in "early disease" is often reported to have clear advantages over ^{18}F-fluoride. However, little has been published comparing ^{18}F-labeled NaF and FDG or other PET radiopharmaceuticals. FDG usually was more likely to detect bone marrow metastases or small osteolytic lesions, presumably lesions with little or no increase in cortical bone turnover. ^{18}F-Labeled NaF was more likely to detect skeletal metastases of tumors that typically have low FDG avidity, such as thyroid cancer or renal cell cancer.[23] For most tumors the sensitivity of FDG in detecting bone metastases seems to be similar to BS; in addition it can be used to monitor the response to chemotherapy and hormonal therapy.[23] The proposed approach by Hoegerle and colleagues[24] for combined administration of FDG and ^{18}F-labeled NaF for cancer imaging has not been widely adopted. In a recent study in 126 patients with lung cancer comparing ^{99m}Tc-MDP planar BS, ^{18}F-fluoride PET, and FDG PET/CT, the investigators showed that FDG PET/CT detected more bone metastases (50) compared with ^{18}F-fluoride PET (40), and in one patient 1 osteolytic bone metastasis was false negative on ^{18}F-fluoride PET, so that it was concluded that PET/CT may obviate the need to perform additional bone scans or ^{18}F-fluoride PET in the staging of nonsmall-cell lung cancer.[25]

In a prospective study of Beheshti and colleagues[26] comparing the value of ^{18}F-fluorocholine (FCH) and ^{18}F-fluoride PET/CT for detection of bony metastases from prostate cancer,

[18]F-fluoride PET/CT demonstrated a higher sensitivity than FCH PET/CT (81% vs 74%).

Interesting is the observation of Wade and colleagues,[27] who described a flare response similar to bone scanning with bisphosphonates and an increase in bone repair after successful treatment of metastasis on the ^{18}F-fluoride study, whereas correlative imaging findings showed a decreased metabolic activity of FDG, which was confirmed by anatomic information provided by CT (sclerosis) and MRI (decreased interval enhancement).

There are several studies that point out the role of static ^{18}F-fluoride PET imaging also in benign skeletal diseases. Similar to BS, ^{18}F-fluoride PET has been performed in patients with low back pain, in which the high resolution of PET imaging achieved detection of various bone anomalies in 55% of the patients.[28] Furthermore, ^{18}F-fluoride PET has been reported to have clinical significance in other benign indications such as early diagnosis of aseptic loosening of knee arthroplasty,[29] and analogous to bone scintigraphy has been used to detect child abuse.[30]

QUANTITATIVE ^{18}F-FLUORIDE PET: METHODOLOGICAL CONSIDERATIONS

The first method for quantitative assessment of bone metabolism by ^{18}F-fluoride in dynamic PET scans was introduced by Hawkins and colleagues[31] in 1992, who introduced a 4-parameter, 3-compartment model for the kinetics of ^{18}F-fluoride in bone (**Fig. 2**). In reflecting the physiologic process, the model describes fluoride transport between plasma and the compartment of free/unmetabolized ^{18}F-fluoride in bone tissue (unbound compartment), and then ionic exchange of the fluoride with hydroxyl groups in hydroxyapatite to form fluoroapatite (bound compartment). The rate constants K_1 and k_2 describe the forward transport from plasma to the unbound bone compartment and the clearance of unmetabolized ^{18}F-fluoride from tissue, respectively. The rate constant k_3 describes binding to bone apatite, and k_4 describes release from the

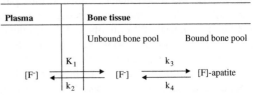

Fig. 2. Three-compartment, 4-parameter model for fluoride bone metabolism.

mineral bone compartment. Quantitative estimates of the rate constants can be obtained by nonlinear regression to the model of tissue time-activity curves obtained by dynamic PET acquisition protocols and the plasma time-activity curve, the so-called input function, obtained by arterial blood sampling and well-counter measurements of the blood samples. From the rate constants one can compute the net fluoride influx rate K, which characterizes fluoride metabolism[9,31–37]: the net rate of fluoride use is obtained by multiplying the plasma concentration of fluoride with K. The fluoride bone influx rate K_{NLR} (mL/min/mL) is the net forward transport parameter and can be calculated as

$$K_{NLR} = K_1 \times k_3/(k_2+k_3)$$

The rate constant K_1 depends on perfusion. For tracers with 100% single-pass extraction, K_1 is equal to the perfusion.

Assuming that the release from the mineral bone compartment is slow, that is, can be neglected for the time period of the dynamic PET sequence (k_4 = 0), the bone influx rate K can also be estimated directly by Patlak graphical analysis.[31,37–40] The single rate constants cannot be calculated by this approach. Patlak analysis involves *linear* regression and, therefore, provides more robust results than *nonlinear* regression methods, which are much more sensitive to the statistical noise in the PET data. Patlak analysis is easily applied not only on the basis of regions of interest but also on the level of voxels. Hawkins and colleagues[31] showed that estimates of the influx rate for fluoride in bone from Patlak graphical analysis are in very good agreement with estimates from nonlinear regression.

These data were confirmed by a study conducted by the authors' group that investigated the relationship of ^{18}F-fluoride bone metabolism estimated with nonlinear regression (NLR), Patlak analysis, and the standardized uptake value (SUV), in patients after resection of a bone tumor, measuring fluoride uptake of the bone graft, the contralateral normal side, and the spine.[41] The SUV is the most widely used parameter for semi-quantification of PET studies in clinical routine. The SUV represents the tracer concentration within a region of interest (ROI)[26] at a given time point, corrected for the injected tracer activity and for patient weight or lean body mass or body surface area.[42] The SUV is easily computed from a single static PET image. Dynamic imaging and blood sampling are not required. In the study by Brenner and colleagues,[41] the ^{18}F-fluoride input rate as well as its changes were strongly correlated between Patlak analysis (K_{Pat}) and NLR (K_{NLR}) (**Fig. 3**). K_{NLR} ranged from 0.0027 to 0.0737 mL/min/mL in a wide variety of bone conditions. ^{18}F-Fluoride flux values obtained by Patlak analysis were almost identical, with a highly significant positive linear correlation (see **Fig. 3**). However, K_{NLR} were higher than K_{Pat} in this study, in agreement with the literature.[31,37,38] The mean difference between K_{NLR} and K_{Pat} was 7%, with a slope of 1.07 for the regression line (K_{NLR} = 1.0731 K_{Pat}; r = 0.99; $P<.01$). This result was explained by the contribution of k_4, which was not completely negligible in this study (range: 0–0.0256 per minute).[41] SUV also showed good correlation with K_{Pat} (r = 0.95) and K_{NLR} (r = 0.93) (**Figs. 4** and **5**). However, in low-uptake areas such as limb bones, SUV analysis was limited by a significantly decreased stability (increased test-retest variability). It was estimated that disease-related or treatment-related changes in fluoride uptake need to be greater than 50% to be detected reliably by SUV analysis, whereas changes in the fluoride influx rate of more than 25% within 6 months could be considered true changes in case of K_{Pat} and K_{NLR}. This result was explained by the fact that especially in low-uptake areas, such as limb bones, relatively a greater fraction of the measured total activity within the ROI is due to blood activity and unbound ^{18}F-fluoride and, thus, is subject to nonbone related effects that increase the variability in repeated measurements. Thus, Brenner and colleagues[41] concluded that SUV is valuable only for high-uptake areas such as the spine or bone metabolic conditions with

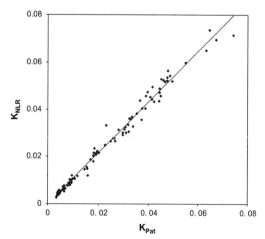

Fig. 3. Positive linear correlation of K_{Pat} (mL/min/mL) and K_{NLR} (mL/min/mL) for ^{18}F-fluoride in both normal and pathologic bone conditions (K_{NLR} = 1.0731 K_{Pat}; r = 0.99; $P<.01$). (*From* Brenner W, Vernon C, Muzi M, et al. Comparison of different quantitative approaches to ^{18}F-fluoride PET scans. J Nucl Med 2004;45(9): 1493–500; with permission.)

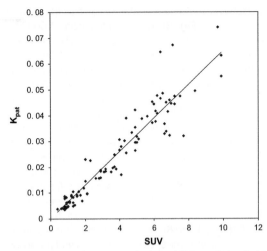

Fig. 4. Positive linear correlation of SUV and K_{Pat} (mL/min/mL) for ^{18}F-fluoride in both normal and pathologic bone conditions (K_{Pat} = 0.0065 SUV; r = 0.95; P<.01). (*From* Brenner W, Vernon C, Muzi M, et al. Comparison of different quantitative approaches to ^{18}F-fluoride PET scans. J Nucl Med 2004;45(9):1493–500; with permission.)

pathophysiologically high fluoride uptake, whereas SUV cannot be recommended to monitor metabolic changes in low-uptake areas such as limb bones.

In another study by the authors' group assessing the metabolic activity of bone grafts, both Patlak-derived bone influx of ^{18}F-fluoride and SUV

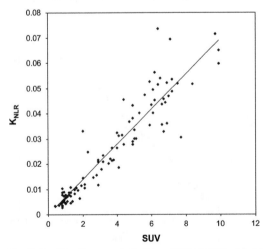

Fig. 5. Positive linear correlation of SUV and K_{NLR} (mL/min/mL) for ^{18}F-fluoride in both normal and pathologic bone conditions (K_{NLR} = 0.0070 SUV; r = 0.93; P<.01). (*From* Brenner W, Vernon C, Muzi M, et al. Comparison of different quantitative approaches to ^{18}F-fluoride PET scans. J Nucl Med 2004;45(9):1493–500; with permission.)

were also found to be strongly correlated with K_{NLR} for baseline values as well as percentage changes over time.[43] Applying a threshold of 20% to consider changes as significant, SUV yielded discrepant results in 5 out of 18 grafts while Patlak findings were identical to NLR. These results again indicate that SUV is less reliable than compartmental approaches.

Frost and colleagues[44] recently compared 4 different quantitative methods for analyzing ^{18}F-fluoride PET of the lumbar spine in 16 patients with osteoporosis at baseline and 6 months later, to evaluate the long-term precision of skeletal kinetic parameters. The imaging results were correlated with biochemical markers of bone formation and bone resorption. The investigators used (1) a 3-compartment model with 4 parameters (K_{4k}), (2) a 3-compartment model with 3 parameters (K_{3k}) assuming k_4 = 0, and (3) Patlak graphical analysis (K_{Pat}) and SUV.[44] The precision of ^{18}F-fluoride PET expressed as coefficient of variation (CV with 95% confidence interval), assessed over 6 months, ranged from 12.2% (9%–19%) for K_{3k}, 13.8% (10%–22%) for K_{Pat}, 14.4% (11%–22%) for SUV, and 26.6% (19%–40%) for K_{4k}. In this study the best precision, shown by the smaller CV and 95% confidence intervals, was found for the 3-compartment model with 3 parameters (K_{3k}). No significant differences in precision were found between SUV, K_{3k}, and K_{Pat}. Moreover, the level of agreement between repeated measurements expressed as an interclass correlation was good for the biochemical markers and for K_{3k} (r = 0.85) and K_{Pat} (r = 0.70), whereas the agreement between repeated measures of K_{4k} was found to be weak (r = 0.44), and no significant correlation was observed for repeated SUV measurements (r = 0.36). Frost and colleagues reported that the most preferred method for quantification, published by Hawkins in 1992, using the 4-parameter, 3-compartment model showed precision errors in their current study of more than double those observed for K_{3k}. The investigators therefore assumed that the inclusion of k_4 in the model would likely have an unfavorable effect on the overall precision of the macroparameter K. The assumption of a zero value for k_4 seemed to increase the precision for estimations of the influx rate K.[44]

There is only one previous study by Brenner and colleagues[41] examining the precision and reproducibility of ^{18}F-fluoride PET. The study compared the quantitative results obtained in 8 normal limb bones and 3 thoracic vertebrae in 8 patients imaged twice within 5 to 7 months, without bone metabolic relevant treatment between the 2 scans.

In the spine, a within-subjects coefficient of variation ranging from 8.8% for SUV to 13.9% for NLR was found. The 95% range of normal change, that is, the range of spontaneous bone metabolic fluctuations plus measurement error, was ±8.6% for SUV, ±7.6% for K_{Pat}, and ±19.6% for K_{NLR}. These findings are well in line with the results of Frost and colleagues[44] obtained in the lumbar spine. For normal limb bones, however, much lower metabolic values were observed by all 3 methods. Consequently, due to a lower signal-to-noise ratio, the 95% range of normal change plus measurement errors within 6 months was ±58.0% for SUV, ±23.0% for Patlak, and ±20.2% for NLR, showing a particularly high variability in SUV repeated measurements and a lower variability for NLR. These findings confirm the suggestion that metabolic changes indicated by SUV in normal- to high-uptake areas such as the spine have similar clinical importance as changes observed by K_{NLR} or Patlak analysis. The limitations of SUV, however, become eminent in low-uptake areas where a significant increase of the variability in repeated measurements was observed, rendering SUV an almost useless parameter.[41]

In accordance to these findings, Frost and colleagues[44] reported that although the precision of SUV was similar to the precision of kinetic parameters and the biochemical markers, repeated measures of SUV values at baseline and at 6 months were not significantly correlated, whereas there was a significant correlation of both the kinetic parameters and the biochemical markers at baseline and 6 months later.

There are still not many studies that have assessed the accuracy of SUV as an estimate of bone metabolism. As already demonstrated, SUV showed a significant linear correlation with modeled influx parameters and seemed to correlate with changes in these parameters in response to bisphosphonate therapy in patients with Paget disease, a condition principally defined by a high ^{18}F-fluoride uptake and, thus, less susceptible to the methodological limitations of SUV.[45] However, further studies are required to prove the accuracy of SUV measurements in quantifying bone metabolism in different pathophysiological settings.

CLINICAL ROLE OF QUANTITATIVE DYNAMIC ^{18}F-FLUORIDE PET

There are several different techniques for assessment of bone turnover. The most direct, but invasive and painful method is histomorphometric analysis of bone biopsies, usually obtained from the iliac crest, which allow evaluation of the integrity of trabecular bone, as well as dynamic measurements of the rates of change at bones surfaces using tetracycline labeling. Another method is the measurement of biochemical markers of bone resorption and bone formation in serum or urine, which is limited by poor precision because of daily variations in bone metabolism of individual patients.[46] Another limitation of serum or urine markers is that these markers represent total bone turnover and do not allow any conclusions on local bone conditions or local changes. Longitudinal assessment of the bone density at sites such as the spine and the hip is also widely used; however, it may take a year before statistically significant changes can be measured in an individual patient.[47] Quantitative ^{18}F-fluoride PET has been shown to be a valuable clinical method for direct noninvasive assessment of bone turnover at clinically important skeletal sites, and is proven to correlate with bone histomorphometry.[37] There are some mostly benign metabolic bone diseases in which the measurement of the kinetics of fluoride ion has been used for characterization of bone metabolism and monitoring response to therapy. ^{18}F-Fluoride PET has been used for characterization of pathologic bone conditions in metabolic bone diseases such as Morbus Paget, osteoporosis, renal osteodystrophy, and for assessment of the viability of bone grafts, fracture healing, and diagnosis of osteonecrosis.[38,39,43–45,48–54] ^{18}F-Fluoride PET offers a *noninvasive* approach for quantitative measurement of bone metabolism and, in comparison with biochemical blood markers, provides localization to specific skeletal sites. Moreover, quantitative imaging results with ^{18}F-fluoride PET have been validated by direct comparison with the gold standard bone biopsy.

In a patient study by Messa and colleagues,[55] the bone metabolic activity measured with ^{18}F-fluoride PET in patients with renal osteodystrophy was correlated with bone histomorphometry. Both the 3-compartment model and Patlak graphical analysis provided quantitative estimates of bone cell activity that correlated with the histomorphometric data. In another experimental study by Piert and colleagues[37] it was shown that ^{18}F-fluoride PET provides quantitative estimates of bone blood flow and metabolic activity that correlate with histomorphometric indices of bone formation in normal bone tissue of the mini pig. Iliac crest bone biopsies were performed immediately before the PET scan to determine static and dynamic indices of bone metabolism (ie, the mineral apposition rate) by bone histomorphometry. A rate constant describing the net forward transport rate of fluoride (K_i) and the fluoride volume flux (K_{flux}) derived from a 2-tissue 3-compartment model was calculated and compared with the results of Patlak graphic analysis (K_{Pat}). A significant correlation was found between the mineral apposition rate and K_i, K_{flux}, K_{Pat}, K_1, and blood flow estimates. Therefore, ^{18}F-fluoride PET seemed a valuable tool that may allow reduction of the number of invasive bone biopsies, facilitating the follow-up of patients with metabolic bone diseases.

Piert and colleagues[56] showed in a preclinical study in mini pigs with parathyroid hormone–related high-turnover bone disease after gastrectomy that bone metabolism assessed with ^{18}F-fluoride PET was significantly increased, but bone blood flow, derived from permeability-surface area product corrected K_1 values, was not. Because bone blood flow and metabolism are coupled in normal bone tissue, the question arose as to whether the capillary permeability and/or surface area might be altered in high-turnover bone disease. Piert and colleagues[56] also measured the bone blood flow in vertebral bodies by dynamic ^{15}O-H_2O PET, followed by dynamic ^{18}F-fluoride PET. The results revealed a significant elevation of K_i and k_3, which was mainly caused by an increase of the fraction of bound tracer in tissue. By contrast, blood flow parameters remained unchanged. Thus, the increased bone metabolism in high-turnover bone disease was found to be mainly related to an upregulation of the amount of ionic exchange of ^{18}F-fluoride with the bone matrix, while tracer delivery remained unchanged.

Several works by Frost and colleagues[44,52–54] investigated the diagnostic potential of ^{18}F-fluoride PET for diagnosis and treatment monitoring of osteoporosis. In a study of 43 women with osteoporosis, 21 of whom received treatment, it was shown that the relationship between regional bone turnover measured with ^{18}F-fluoride PET and changes in bone mineral density (BMD) was equivalent to that seen for biochemical markers for bone formation and bone resorption. Treated women in the highest tertile of bone turnover, measured both with ^{18}F-fluoride PET and biochemical markers, showed the greatest annual percentage increase in BMD in the lumbar spine. The annual increase in lumbar spine BMD was 1.8%, 2.2%, and 3.2% for women in the lowest, middle, and highest tertile of biochemical markers, respectively, which was similar to that obtained for the regional measurement of K_i with 1.7%, 2.2%, and 2.7%, respectively. Vice versa, untreated women in the highest tertile of regional and global bone turnover had larger decreases in lumbar spine BMD compared with those in the lowest tertile. The study was a demonstration of the relationship between regional bone turnover measured

directly with ^{18}F-fluoride PET and changes in BMD and biochemical markers, indicating ^{18}F-fluoride PET as a reliable method for monitoring patients with osteoporosis.[54] In a further study the same investigators elaborated the heterogeneity in terms of bone perfusion and turnover in different skeletal sites in treatment-naïve and treated postmenopausal women measured with ^{18}F-fluoride PET.[52] In proportion of trabecular and cortical bone sites, significant differences were observed for the bone perfusion (K_1), bone turnover (K_i), and the rate constant k_2 (measuring the reverse transport) between the lumbar spine and the humerus, all of the constants being higher in the lumbar spine. The ratio K_i/K_1 describing the unidirectional extraction efficiency to bone mineral was significantly greater in the humerus than in the lumbar spine. In a previous study by Cook and colleagues,[32] similar regional differences in ^{18}F-fluoride kinetics were observed between the lumbar spine and the humerus in postmenopausal women using 3-compartmental modeling. These observations allow some better understanding of the differences of pathophysiology of metabolic impairment in different skeletal regions as well as the regional differences in response to treatment. Frost and colleagues[53] also investigated the effect of risedronate on bone metabolism at the lumbar spine using ^{18}F-fluoride PET at baseline and after 6 months of therapy in 18 women with osteoporosis. Mean vertebral K_i decreased significantly by 18.4% from baseline to 6 months post treatment. This percentage decrease was similar in magnitude to the decrease observed for bone-specific alkaline phosphatase, a marker of bone formation. There were no significant differences in K_1, k_3, and k_4, but there was a significant increase in k_2, reflecting an increasing reverse transport of fluoride from the extravascular tissue compartment to plasma from baseline to 6 months after treatment. There was also a significant decrease from baseline to 6 months in the fraction of tracer in the extravascular tissue space that underwent specific binding to the bone matrix ($k_3/[k_2 + k_3]$), decreasing by 18.1%. This study for the first time showed a direct metabolic effect of antiresorptive treatment on skeletal kinetics at the clinically important site of the lumbar spine.

Another clinical indication of quantitative PET imaging has been the assessment of the time course of graft healing in allogeneic bone grafts of the limbs after surgery. To evaluate bone graft healing during follow-up, clinical examinations and radiography are the most widely used and accepted tools. However, plain radiography is unreliable in early prediction of impaired graft healing because it assesses morphologic signs such as gaps at junction sites, callus formation, and bridging bone formation, which occur late in the normal course of healing. Because other imaging techniques such as CT, MRI, or BS are even less accepted or standardized, imaging assessments for bone allografts are controversial. ^{18}F-Fluoride PET has the potential to exactly measure fluoride bone metabolism in specific spatial regions. The authors therefore performed a total of 52 dynamic ^{18}F-fluoride PET studies in 34 patients with cancellous and full bone grafts.[43] Metabolic bone activity in cancellous grafts decreased by 25% from 6 to 12 months post surgery, and revealed a total decrease of 65% after 2 years for SUV, Patlak, and NLR. Full bone grafts showed first an increase by 20% from 6 to 12 months, and decreased from then on to 70% of the initial activity at the end of 2 years by either quantification method. In 2 patients with nonunion of their full bone grafts an increase of SUV, K_{Pat}, K_{NLR}, and K_1 far above average and outside the normal time pattern was observed. Thus, quantitative ^{18}F-fluoride PET was shown to be a useful tool for the assessment of metabolic activity and normal healing in bone grafts of the limbs. Some other groups showed similar results using ^{18}F-fluoride PET after skeletal surgery. Piert and colleagues[39] also observed an increased bone activity after a mean follow-up of 2 years after hip augmentation surgery with cancellous grafts, and explained these findings with continued stress to the normal surrounding bone. Differing results were reported by the group of Berding and colleagues[48]: 6 months after oral surgery with transplantation of vascularized fibula grafts, K_{NLR} values were returned to the level of the reference region in the cervical spine. The most likely explanation for these findings is that K_{NLR} values in limb bones are significantly lower with a mean of 0.0081 ± 0.0048 mL/min/mL compared with values for the cervical spine of 0.0508 ± 0.0193 mL/min/mL.[49] Metabolic values in fibula grafts similar to the cervical spine therefore would still indicate an increased bone metabolism because K_i values in normal limb bones are significantly lower than in the spine, as observed by both Piert and colleagues[39] and Brenner and colleagues.[43] In another study on fibula grafts used for mandibular reconstruction, the same group hypothesized that normal healing is characterized by low osteoblastic activity and increased perfusion. Dynamic measurements in 11 patients early and late after surgery showed that K_1, but not K_i was increased in uncomplicated cases after surgery, while patients with graft necroses showed a markedly reduced ^{18}F-fluoride influx.[48] In a similar study of 5 patients with femoral allografts inserted for treatment of prosthetic loosening, quantitative ^{18}F-fluoride PET showed increased uptake during

the first year. Six years after surgery, the ^{18}F-fluoride uptake normalized compared with the contralateral femur indicating full regeneration.[57]

Several publications showed the role of quantitative ^{18}F-fluoride PET in the management of patients with Paget disease, a metabolic bone disorder characterized with accelerated bone turnover.[45,50] Installe and colleagues[45] were able to demonstrate that ^{18}F-fluoride PET was a useful tool for monitoring response to treatment with bisphosphonates in pagetic patients. One month after initiation of treatment, a significant decrease of ^{18}F-fluoride uptake by approximately 30% was observed measured with K_{Pat}, K_{NLR}, and SUV, and after 6 months of treatment ^{18}F-fluoride uptake diminished further by 23% to 26%. Furthermore, the study showed that SUV and changes in SUV correlated with K_{Pat} and K_{NLR} and changes thereof, suggesting that simple static acquisition and SUV measurement might be used for monitoring response to treatment with bisphosphonates in patients with Paget disease. Again, one should note that SUV seems to be a reliable measure only in bone conditions with high fluoride uptake such as Paget disease.

SUMMARY

This article reviews the role of ^{18}F-fluoride PET in the skeleton, with a focus on (1) the underlying physiologic and pathophysiological processes of various different conditions of bone metabolism and (2) methodological aspects of quantitative measurement of ^{18}F-fluoride kinetics. To date, several reports on fluoride PET are available on both benign and malignant diseases. Recent comparative studies have demonstrated that ^{18}F-fluoride PET and, to an even greater extent, PET/CT are more accurate than ^{99m}Tc-bisphosphonate SPECT for identifying malignant and benign lesions of the skeleton. In these studies, the bone agent ^{18}F-fluoride has been mainly used to evaluate bone metastases qualitatively. There are also many reports on several focal and systemic skeletal disorders and metabolic conditions, for example, osteoporosis and Paget disease, healing of bone grafts, or on monitoring bone-relevant treatment, in which ^{18}F-fluoride has been used applying standard (semi-) quantitative approaches including compartment modeling by nonlinear regression, Patlak analysis, and SUV.

REFERENCES

1. Blau M, Nagler W, Bender MA. A new isotope for bone scanning. J Nucl Med 1962;3:332–4.

2. Subramanian G, McAfee JG, Bell EG, et al. 99m Tc-labeled polyphosphate as a skeletal imaging agent. Radiology 1972;102(3):701–4.

3. Subramanian G, McAfee JG, Blair RJ, et al. Technetium-99m-labeled stannous imidodiphosphate, a new radiodiagnostic agent for bone scanning: comparison with other ^{99m}Tc complexes. J Nucl Med 1975;16(12):1137–43.

4. Grant FD, Fahey FH, Packard AB, et al. Skeletal PET with ^{18}F-fluoride: applying new technology to an old tracer. J Nucl Med 2008;49(1):68–78.

5. Dahlbom M, Hoffman EJ, Hoh CK, et al. Whole-body positron emission tomography: part I. Methods and performance characteristics. J Nucl Med 1992; 33(6):1191–9.

6. DeGrado TR, Turkington TG, Williams JJ, et al. Performance characteristics of a whole-body PET scanner. J Nucl Med 1994;35(8):1398–406.

7. Caverzasio J, Palmer G, Bonjour JP. Fluoride: mode of action. Bone 1998;22(6):585–9.

8. Krishnamurthy GT, Huebotter RJ, Tubis M, et al. Pharmaco-kinetics of current skeletal-seeking radiopharmaceuticals. AJR Am J Roentgenol 1976; 126(2):293–301.

9. Wootton R, Dore C. The single-passage extraction of ^{18}F in rabbit bone. Clin Phys Physiol Meas 1986; 7(4):333–43.

10. Costeas A, Woodard HQ, Laughlin JS. Depletion of ^{18}F from blood flowing through bone. J Nucl Med 1970;11(1):43–5.

11. Blake GM, Park-Holohan SJ, Cook GJ, et al. Quantitative studies of bone with the use of 18F-fluoride and ^{99m}Tc-methylene diphosphonate. Semin Nucl Med 2001;31(1):28–49.

12. Tosteson D. Halide transport in red blood cells. Acta Physiol Scand 1959;46:19–41.

13. Hyldstrup L, McNair P, Ring P, et al. Studies on diphosphonate kinetics. Part II: whole body bone uptake rate during constant infusion—a refined index of bone metabolism. Eur J Nucl Med 1987; 12(12):585–8.

14. Hyldstrup L, McNair P, Ring P, et al. Studies on diphosphonate kinetics. Part I: evaluation of plasma elimination curves during 24 h. Eur J Nucl Med 1987;12(12):581–4.

15. Park-Holohan SJ, Blake GM, Fogelman I. Quantitative studies of bone using (18)F-fluoride and (99m)Tc-methylene diphosphonate: evaluation of renal and whole-blood kinetics. Nucl Med Commun 2001;22(9):1037–44.

16. Petren-Mallmin M, Andreasson I, Ljunggren O, et al. Skeletal metastases from breast cancer: uptake of ^{18}F-fluoride measured with positron emission tomography in correlation with CT. Skeletal Radiol 1998; 27(2):72–6.

17. Schirrmeister H, Guhlmann A, Elsner K, et al. Sensitivity in detecting osseous lesions depends on anatomic localization: planar bone scintigraphy versus ^{18}F PET. J Nucl Med 1999;40(10): 1623–9.

18. Schirrmeister H, Glatting G, Hetzel J, et al. Prospective evaluation of the clinical value of planar bone scans, SPECT, and (18)F-labeled NaF PET in newly diagnosed lung cancer. J Nucl Med 2001;42(12): 1800–4.

19. Schirrmeister H, Kotzerke J, Rentschler M, et al. [Positron-emission tomography of the skeletal system using ^{18}FNa: the incidence, pattern of the findings and distribution of benign changes]. Rofo 1998;169(3):310–4 [in German].

20. Schirrmeister H, Rentschler M, Kotzerke J, et al. [Imaging of the normal skeletal system with ^{18}F Na-PET compared with conventional skeletal scintigraphy using Tc99m-MDP]. Rofo 1998;168(5):451–6 [in German].

21. Even-Sapir E, Metser U, Flusser G, et al. Assessment of malignant skeletal disease: initial experience with ^{18}F-fluoride PET/CT and comparison between ^{18}F-fluoride PET and ^{18}F-fluoride PET/CT. J Nucl Med 2004;45(2):272–8.

22. Even-Sapir E, Metser U, Mishani E, et al. The detection of bone metastases in patients with high-risk prostate cancer: ^{99m}Tc-MDP planar bone scintigraphy, single- and multi-field-of-view SPECT, ^{18}F-fluoride PET, and ^{18}F-fluoride PET/CT. J Nucl Med 2006;47(2):287–97.

23. Langsteger W, Heinisch M, Fogelman I. The role of fluorodeoxyglucose, ^{18}F-dihydroxyphenylalanine, ^{18}F-choline, and ^{18}F-fluoride in bone imaging with emphasis on prostate and breast. Semin Nucl Med 2006;36(1):73–92.

24. Hoegerle S, Juengling F, Otte A, et al. Combined FDG and [F-18]fluoride whole-body PET: a feasible two-in-one approach to cancer imaging? Radiology 1998;209(1):253–8.

25. Kruger S, Buck AK, Mottaghy FM, et al. Detection of bone metastases in patients with lung cancer: ^{99m}Tc-MDP planar bone scintigraphy, ^{18}F-fluoride PET or ^{18}F-FDG PET/CT. Eur J Nucl Med Mol Imaging 2009;36(11):1807–12.

26. Beheshti M, Vali R, Waldenberger P, et al. Detection of bone metastases in patients with prostate cancer by ^{18}F fluorocholine and ^{18}F fluoride PET-CT: a comparative study. Eur J Nucl Med Mol Imaging 2008;35(10):1766–74.

27. Wade AA, Scott JA, Kuter I, et al. Flare response in ^{18}F-fluoride ion PET bone scanning. AJR Am J Roentgenol 2006;186(6):1783–6.

28. Lim R, Fahey FH, Drubach LA, et al. Early experience with fluorine-18 sodium fluoride bone PET in young patients with back pain. J Pediatr Orthop 2007;27(3):277–82.

29. Sterner T, Pink R, Freudenberg L, et al. The role of [18F]fluoride positron emission tomography in the

early detection of aseptic loosening of total knee arthroplasty. Int J Surg 2007;5(2):99–104.

30. Drubach LA, Sapp MV, Laffin S, et al. Fluorine-18 NaF PET imaging of child abuse. Pediatr Radiol 2008;38(7):776–9.

31. Hawkins RA, Choi Y, Huang SC, et al. Evaluation of the skeletal kinetics of fluorine-18-fluoride ion with PET. J Nucl Med 1992;33(5):633–42.

32. Cook GJ, Lodge MA, Blake GM, et al. Differences in skeletal kinetics between vertebral and humeral bone measured by ^{18}F-fluoride positron emission tomography in postmenopausal women. J Bone Miner Res 2000;15(4):763–9.

33. Garnett ES, Bowen BM, Coates G, et al. An analysis of factors which influence the local accumulation of bone- seeking radiopharmaceuticals. Invest Radiol 1975;10(6):564–8.

34. Green JR, Reeve J, Tellez M, et al. Skeletal blood flow in metabolic disorders of the skeleton. Bone 1987;8(5):293–7.

35. Hoh CK, Hawkins RA, Dahlbom M, et al. Whole body skeletal imaging with [18F]fluoride ion and PET. J Comput Assist Tomogr 1993;17(1):34–41.

36. Nahmias C, Cockshott WP, Belbeck LW, et al. Measurement of absolute bone blood flow by positron emission tomography. Skeletal Radiol 1986;15(3):198–200.

37. Piert M, Zittel TT, Becker GA, et al. Assessment of porcine bone metabolism by dynamic [18F]fluoride ion PET: correlation with bone histomorphometry. J Nucl Med 2001;42(7):1091–100.

38. Berding G, Burchert W, van den Hoff J, et al. Evaluation of the incorporation of bone grafts used in maxillofacial surgery with [18F]fluoride ion and dynamic positron emission tomography. Eur J Nucl Med 1995;22(10):1133–40.

39. Piert M, Winter E, Becker GA, et al. Allogenic bone graft viability after hip revision arthroplasty assessed by dynamic [18F]fluoride ion positron emission tomography. Eur J Nucl Med 1999;26(6):615–24.

40. Patlak CS, Blasberg RG, Fenstermacher JD. Graphical evaluation of blood-to-brain transfer constants from multiple- time uptake data. J Cereb Blood Flow Metab 1983;3(1):1–7.

41. Brenner W, Vernon C, Muzi M, et al. Comparison of different quantitative approaches to ^{18}F-fluoride PET scans. J Nucl Med 2004;45(9):1493–500.

42. Weber WA, Ziegler SI, Thodtmann R, et al. Reproducibility of metabolic measurements in malignant tumors using FDG PET. J Nucl Med 1999;40:1771–7.

43. Brenner W, Vernon C, Conrad EU, et al. Assessment of the metabolic activity of bone grafts with (18)F-fluoride PET. Eur J Nucl Med Mol Imaging 2004; 31(9):1291–8.

44. Frost ML, Blake GM, Park-Holohan SJ, et al. Long-term precision of ^{18}F-fluoride PET skeletal kinetic

studies in the assessment of bone metabolism. J Nucl Med 2008;49(5):700–7.

45. Installe J, Nzeusseu A, Bol A, et al. (18)F-fluoride PET for monitoring therapeutic response in Paget's disease of bone. J Nucl Med 2005;46(10):1650–8.

46. Looker AC, Bauer DC, Chesnut CH 3rd, et al. Clinical use of biochemical markers of bone remodeling: current status and future directions. Osteoporos Int 2000;11(6):467–80.

47. Eastell R. Treatment of postmenopausal osteoporosis. N Engl J Med 1998;338(11):736–46.

48. Berding G, Schliephake H, van den Hoff J, et al. Assessment of the incorporation of revascularized fibula grafts used for mandibular reconstruction with F-18-PET. Nuklearmedizin 2001;40(2):51–8.

49. Blake GM, Park-Holohan SJ, Fogelman I. Quantitative studies of bone in postmenopausal women using (18)F-fluoride and (99m)Tc-methylene diphosphonate. J Nucl Med 2002;43(3):338–45.

50. Cook GJ, Blake GM, Marsden PK, et al. Quantification of skeletal kinetic indices in Paget's disease using dynamic ^{18}F-fluoride positron emission tomography. J Bone Miner Res 2002;17(5):854–9.

51. Cook GJ, Maisey MN, Fogelman I. Fluorine-18-FDG PET in Paget's disease of bone. J Nucl Med 1997; 38(9):1495–7.

52. Frost ML, Blake GM, Cook GJ, et al. Differences in regional bone perfusion and turnover between lumbar spine and distal humerus: (18)F-fluoride PET study of treatment-naïve and treated postmenopausal women. Bone 2009;45(5):942–8.

53. Frost ML, Cook GJ, Blake GM, et al. A prospective study of risedronate on regional bone metabolism and blood flow at the lumbar spine measured by ^{18}F-fluoride positron emission tomography. J Bone Miner Res 2003;18(12):2215–22.

54. Frost ML, Cook GJ, Blake GM, et al. The relationship between regional bone turnover measured using ^{18}F-fluoride positron emission tomography and changes in BMD is equivalent to that seen for biochemical markers of bone turnover. J Clin Densitom 2007;10(1):46–54.

55. Messa C, Goodman WG, Hoh CK, et al. Bone metabolic activity measured with positron emission tomography and [18F]fluoride ion in renal osteodystrophy: correlation with bone histomorphometry. J Clin Endocrinol Metab 1993;77(4):949–55.

56. Piert M, Machulla HJ, Jahn M, et al. Coupling of porcine bone blood flow and metabolism in high-turnover bone disease measured by [(15)O]H(2)O and [(18)F]fluoride ion positron emission tomography. Eur J Nucl Med Mol Imaging 2002;29(7):907–14.

57. Ullmark G, Sorensen J, Langstrom B, et al. Bone regeneration 6 years after impaction bone grafting: a PET analysis. Acta Orthop 2007;78(2):201–5.

18F-Fluoride PET in Osteoporosis

Michelle L. Frost, PhD[a], Glen M. Blake, PhD[a,*],
Ignac Fogelman, MD[b]

KEYWORDS

- Osteoporosis • 18F-Fluoride PET
- Bone turnover • Bone perfusion

OSTEOPOROSIS

Osteoporosis is a disease characterized by low bone mass and microarchitectural deterioration of bone tissue, resulting in an increased risk of fracture.[1] The consequences of fracture include chronic pain, disability, a reduced quality of life, and increased mortality.[2] In addition, osteoporosis is associated with a significant economic burden, with costs estimated to be $17.9 billion per year in the United States and £1.7 billion per year in the United Kingdom,[3] and these costs are expected to continue to increase globally.[4] The inverse relationship between bone density and fracture is well known, with patients with lower bone density having a greater risk of fracture.[5] As a consequence of the strength of this relationship, a diagnosis of osteoporosis was until very recently based entirely on measurements of bone mineral density (BMD) by dual x-ray absorptiometry (DXA).[6] Recently, however, there has been a shift of focus from bone density to other factors that contribute to bone strength and fracture risk. This shift is important, as a large proportion of fractures occur in people who would not be classified as osteoporotic according to conventional diagnostic criteria,[7] that is, a BMD value more than 2.5 standard deviations below the young adult normative mean. Clinical risk factures, in particular those that are associated with fracture risk independent of BMD, such as age, maternal history of hip fracture, and corticosteroid use, can be used alone or in combination with a measurement of femoral neck BMD to determine 10-year fracture risk (FRAX score).[8,9] Intervention thresholds and guidelines based on these 10-year fracture risk scores have been published in the United Kingdom to aid in clinical therapeutic decision making.[10]

There has been considerable interest in the role of bone turnover role in the pathophysiology of osteoporosis.[11] Just as for all living tissues, bone is constantly renewing itself by remodeling, whereby bone osteoclasts and osteoblasts undertake the process of bone resorption and bone formation, respectively. This process of remodeling is referred to as the rate of bone turnover, bone remodeling, or bone metabolism, but for the purpose of this review the term bone turnover is used. The effects of therapies, developed for the treatment of osteoporosis, on BMD and fracture risk are mediated through their direct effects on osteoclasts and osteoblasts.[12] The rate of bone turnover is independently associated with fracture risk,[13,14] and large trials of antiresorptive treatments for osteoporosis have shown that changes in bone turnover with treatment are independently associated with changes in fracture risk.[15,16]

MEASUREMENTS OF BONE TURNOVER
Bone Biopsy and Histomorphometry

Unlike techniques for measuring bone density, which are readily available and simple to perform, methods for measuring bone turnover are much more involved, particularly in a clinical setting.

[a] Osteoporosis Unit, King's College London, Guy's Campus, Great Maze Pond, London SE1 9RT, UK
[b] Department of Nuclear Medicine, King's College London, Guy's Campus, Great Maze Pond, London SE1 9RT, UK
* Corresponding author.
E-mail address: glen.blake@kcl.ac.uk

PET Clin 5 (2010) 259–274
doi:10.1016/j.cpet.2010.02.007

The dynamic quantification of bone turnover by tetracycline labeling and bone biopsy at the iliac crest is considered the gold standard for the direct assessment of turnover activity. However, this technique is invasive, is subject to large measurement errors, and involves multiple biopsy specimens to assess changes in response to therapy.[17] Another limitation of this technique is that it is restricted to a single site, the iliac crest, which may not be representative of other important sites within the skeleton such as the spine and hip. In addition, only a few specialist centers are able to perform bone histomorphometry, and it is a complex and costly technique.[18]

Biochemical Markers of Bone Turnover

Although bone biopsy remains the gold standard for quantifying bone turnover, currently the most common and practical method for measuring this is by using biochemical markers of bone turnover.[19,20] Enzymes or bone breakdown products associated with bone resorption or bone formation can be readily measured in urine or serum.[20] These markers have been used effectively to examine the relationship between bone turnover and fracture risk[15,16] and to evaluate the contribution of changes in bone turnover to antifracture efficacy in clinical trials. Although the most practical choice for measuring the rate of bone turnover, particularly in response to therapy, bone markers reflect global skeletal function and cannot provide information on bone turnover at specific sites of the skeleton. Further, it is not possible to differentiate between trabecular and cortical bone or between the axial and appendicular skeleton.[11] It is more informative to examine regional rather than global differences in bone caused by significant variations between skeletal sites in terms of age-related bone loss, disease progression, and response to treatment. The use of biochemical markers in individuals in a clinical setting is also limited because of significant diurnal variation, a lack of appropriate reference ranges, and the need to acquire samples with patients in a fasting state for optimal results.[20]

Radionuclide Measurements of Bone

Quantitative radionuclide measurements of bone using bone tracers such as ^{18}F-fluoride and ^{99m}Tc-methylene diphosphonate allow the noninvasive assessment of bone turnover both globally and at specific sites of the skeleton, including clinically important sites such as the lumbar spine and hip.[21–34] In a review of the role of bone turnover in osteoporosis, which emphasized the importance of bone turnover regarding skeletal fragility and the effects of bone-active agents, Heaney[11] recognized that radionuclide techniques offer the only method by which information about specific skeletal sites can be obtained. In addition to this advantage over conventional methods of allowing an assessment of regional bone turnover, imaging techniques such as ^{18}F-fluoride PET are noninvasive and, unlike bone biopsy, can be readily applied in a clinical setting.

^{18}F-Fluoride PET allows the quantitative assessment of both bone perfusion and osteoblastic activity.[31,32,35,36] ^{18}F-fluoride PET has been used to investigate regional bone turnover in patients with osteoporosis[24,37,38] and other metabolic bone diseases,[22,29,31] as well as the effects of drugs developed for the treatment of these diseases.[23,29,37] ^{18}F-fluoride PET may also have a role in the assessment of bone viability following allogeneic bone grafts and joint replacement (see the article by Apostolova and colleagues elsewhere in this issue for further exploration of this topic).

^{18}F-FLUORIDE

The use of ^{18}F-fluoride for skeletal imaging was first introduced by Blau and colleagues[39] in 1962, well before the arrival of commercial PET scanners. ^{18}F-Fluoride is rapidly cleared from plasma and has a high affinity for bone, resulting in high tissue to background ratios and consequently high-quality images. The ^{18}F-ion exchanges with the hydroxyl groups in hydroxyapatite crystals on the surface of the bone matrix, preferentially at sites of high osteoblastic activity and newly mineralizing bone.[40,41] The ion then migrates into the crystalline matrix of bone where it remains until the bone undergoes remodeling.[42,43] ^{18}F-fluoride is taken up by red blood cells accounting for approximately 30% of the flux in blood.[44] This red cell fluoride appears to be largely available to bone because the single-pass extraction efficiency of ^{18}F-fluoride approaches 100%.[43,45] Unlike the more widely used bone tracer ^{99m}Tc–methyl diphosphonate (^{99m}Tc-MDP), plasma protein binding of ^{18}F-fluoride is minimal,[43] allowing imaging to be performed more quickly following tracer administration compared with ^{99m}Tc-MDP gamma camera imaging.[42] Renal clearance of fluoride as a proportion of glomerular filtration rate is reduced at low urine flow rates, so adequate hydration is important in whole-body fluoride kinetic studies to avoid uncontrolled effects.[43] The primary clinical application of ^{18}F-fluoride PET is oncology for the identification of skeletal lesions, and recent evidence suggests ^{18}F-fluoride PET and hybrid ^{18}F-fluoride PET/computed tomography imaging offers superior sensitivity compared with ^{99m}Tc-MDP planar scintigraphy and single-photon emission computed tomography (SPECT) for the detection of metastatic lesions.[46–49]

SKELETAL KINETIC STUDIES USING 18F-FLUORIDE PET

The use of ^{18}F-fluoride PET for the quantitative assessment of regional bone metabolism was first introduced by Hawkins and colleagues[28] in 1992. Following dynamic PET imaging and measurement of an arterial plasma input function, nonlinear regression analysis using a 3-compartment, 4-parameter model can be applied to derive rate constants describing the transport of fluoride between plasma, an extravascular bone compartment, and bone mineral compartment, as shown in **Fig. 1**. K_1 describes the unidirectional clearance of fluoride from plasma to the whole of the bone tissue, k_2 the reverse transport of fluoride from the extravascular compartment to plasma, and k_3 and k_4 represent the incorporation and release from the bone mineral compartment. Of these rate constants, K_1, the plasma clearance of fluoride to total bone tissue, approximates to the rate of bone perfusion.[35,36] K_i, representing the net clearance of fluoride to the bone mineral compartment, correlates closely with histomorphometric parameters including the bone formation and mineral apposition rate (**Fig. 2**), and therefore provides a quantitative assessment of regional bone turnover.[31,32] K_i is calculated as:

$$K_i = K_1 \times k_3/(k_2+k_3) \ mL.min^{-1}.mL^{-1} \quad (1)$$

The macroparameter K_i can also be calculated by Patlak graphical analysis using a 3-compartment, 3-parameter model. This method assumes that fluoride is irreversibly bound to bone mineral, ie, $k_4 = 0$. Studies have demonstrated a good correlation between these 2 quantitative approaches.[27–29,32]

Both methods described here require dynamic imaging and multiple blood sampling, along with complex computational methods. As typically used for clinical fluorodeoxyglucose (FDG) PET studies, standardized uptake values (SUV) can be calculated providing a semiquantitative measurement of bone turnover. Standardized uptake values represent tissue activity within a region of interest (ROI) corrected for injected activity and patient weight. However, the correlation between SUV and bone histomorphometric parameters obtained using the gold standard of bone biopsy has yet to be reported. The long-term precision of these quantitative and semiquantitative parameters has been examined by Frost and colleagues.[50] Sixteen postmenopausal women with osteoporosis or significant osteopenia underwent ^{18}F-fluoride PET of the lumbar spine on 2 occasions, 6 months apart. Long-term precision of K_i, derived using a 3k 3-compartmental model and Patlak graphical analysis, and SUV was approximately 13% and similar to that observed using the conventional method of biochemical markers measured in the same subjects at the same time points. It was reported that the precision of K_i derived using a 4k-parameter, 3-compartmental model was almost twice that seen for the other parameters, most likely because of the uncertainty in calculating k_4 with only a 1-hour scan acquisition time (**Table 1**).[50] These different quantitative approaches are discussed in more detail (see the article by Apostolova and colleagues elsewhere in this issue for further exploration of this topic).

18F-FLUORIDE PET TO ASSESS BONE TURNOVER IN OSTEOPOROSIS

Recent evidence has established that factors in addition to bone mass, such as bone geometry, microarchitecture, and bone remodeling, are important determinants of fracture risk.[11] It has also been shown that the rate of bone turnover is an independent predictor of fracture risk.[13,14] High bone turnover increases fracture risk and exacerbates bone loss by increasing the remodeling space, creating local foci of structural weakness and in some cases trabecular perforation.[11] Large trials of antiresorptive therapies for

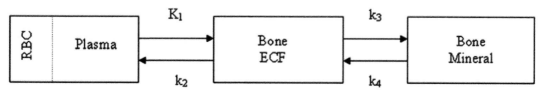

Fig. 1. The 3-compartmental bone kinetic model used by Hawkins and colleagues to analyze PET ^{18}F-fluoride bone studies. See text for description of rate constants. RBC, red blood cells; ECF, bone extracellular fluid space. (*From* Frost ML, Blake GM, Cook GJ, et al. Differences in regional bone perfusion and turnover between lumbar spine and distal humerus: 18F-fluoride PET study of treatment-naïve and treated postmenopausal women. Bone 2009;45:942-8; with permission.)

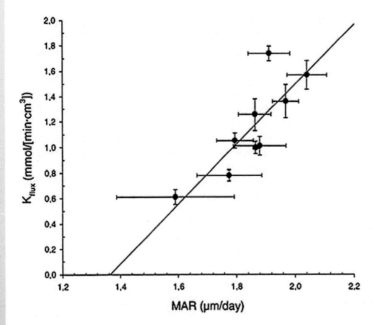

Fig. 2. The correlation between mineral apposition rate (MAR) obtained from iliac crest bone biopsies and fluoride volume flux (K_{flux}) in 9 mini pigs. Data represent mean of 20 sites of each biopsy and 6 regions of interest with their respective standard deviations as error bars in both directions (x- and y-axes). Linear regression analysis yielded a highly significant correlation between these 2 parameters ($r^2 = 0.65$; $y = -3.2 + 2.23x$; $P<.01$). (*From* Piert M, Zittel TT, Becker GA, et al. Assessment of porcine bone metabolism by dynamic ^{18}F-fluoride PET: correlation with bone histomorphometry. J Nucl Med 2001; 42:1091–100; with permission from the Society of Nuclear Medicine.)

osteoporosis have established that changes in turnover correlate with changes in fracture risk independent of BMD.[15,16] A 3-year study of the effects of the antiresorptive agent risedronate demonstrated that changes in bone resorption markers accounted for approximately two-thirds of the drug's effect on reducing the risk of vertebral fracture.[15] The most practical and widely used method for estimating bone turnover in clinical practice is urinary and serum biochemical markers. However, with significant variations between skeletal sites in age-related bone loss, disease progression, and response to treatment, it is more informative to examine regional rather than global differences in bone metabolism, particularly as it allows comparisons to be made between sites with varying amounts of trabecular and cortical bone. As stated previously,

Table 1
Long-term precision of ^{18}F-fluoride PET and biochemical markers measured in 16 postmenopausal women over 6 months

Parameter	RMS SD	CV% (95% CI)	Intraclass Correlation (95% CI)
^{18}F-Fluoride PET			
K_{i-4k} mL min^{-1} mL^{-1}	0.007	26.6 (19.7–41.2)	0.44 (−0.04–0.76)[b]
K_{i-3k} mL min^{-1} mL^{-1}	0.002	12.2 (8.9–18.6)[a]	0.85 (0.5–0.9)[c]
K_{i-PAT} mL min^{-1} mL^{-1}	0.003	13.8 (10.3–21.5)[a]	0.70 (0.33–0.88)[c]
SUV_{mean}	0.775	14.4 (10.6–22.3)	0.36 (−0.16–0.72)
Biochemical markers			
Bone-specific ALP (U/L)	1.81	9.9 (7.3–15.4)	0.87 (0.67–0.95)[c]
Deoxypyridinoline (nmol/mm)	0.87	13.9 (10.3–21.5)	0.76 (0.44–0.91)[c]
Osteocalcin (ng/mL)	1.9	17.8 (13.1–27.5)	0.60 (0.19–0.84)[b]

95% confidence interval (CI) estimated from the χ^2 distribution.
Abbreviations: ALP, alkaline phosphatase; CV, coefficient of variation; K_{i-PAT}, Patlak graphical analysis; K_{i-3k}, 3-compartment 3k model; K_{i-4k}, 3-compartment 4k model; RMS SD, root mean square standard deviation.
[a] $P<.05$ versus K_{i-4k}
[b] $P<0.05$
[c] $P<.001$

Adapted from Frost ML, Blake GM, Park-Holohan SJ, et al. Long-term precision of ^{18}F-Fluoride PET skeletal kinetic studies in the assessment of bone metabolism. J Nucl Med 2008; 49(5):700–7; with permission from the Society of Nuclear Medicine.

quantitative radionuclide measurements, including ^{18}F-fluoride PET, offer the only methodology allowing direct assessment of regional bone turnover at the clinically important fracture sites such as the spine and hip.

Pathophysiology of Osteoporosis

In a study of 72 postmenopausal women, ^{18}F-fluoride PET was used to examine differences in regional bone turnover at the lumbar spine in women with and without osteoporosis.[24] An example of a summed ^{18}F-fluoride PET scan of the lumbar spine is shown in **Fig. 3**. Women were classified as normal, osteopenic, or osteoporotic according to standard BMD diagnostic criteria.[6] The net clearance of fluoride to bone mineral (K_i) was found to be 17% lower at the lumbar spine in the osteoporotic group compared with both the osteopenic and normal groups. K_i was also found to be reduced in a small number of patients with low BMD at the spine.[34] SUV at the lumbar spine have also been reported to be significantly lower in postmenopausal women with osteoporosis than in those with osteopenia.[37] This result is in keeping with those from bone histomorphometric studies that have revealed impaired osteoblastic activity and reduced bone formation at the cellular level with postmenopausal osteoporosis.[17,51–55] Of note, global biochemical markers of bone formation measured in addition to ^{18}F-fluoride PET in the study by Frost and colleagues[24] of 72 postmenopausal women were significantly higher in those with osteoporosis, in contrast to the ^{18}F-fluoride PET results. This finding demonstrates the importance of performing measurements at the regional level, as it is likely that global measurements may mask, exaggerate, or in some cases attenuate what is going on at specific sites of the skeleton. A dynamic ^{18}F-fluoride PET study in a 61-year old female patient with severe osteoporosis and history of multiple fractures as a result of long-term glucocorticoid treatment revealed reduced fluoride influx in nonfractured vertebrae.[38] This finding is consistent with the impairment in osteoblastic function and severely suppressed bone formation in glucocorticoid-induced osteoporosis.[56] ^{18}F-fluoride PET has also been used to investigate the profound bone effects of gastrectomy using a porcine model.[33] In this study, total gastrectomy resulted in significantly increased K_i values (+36%) compared with sham-operated animals and a reduction of BMD of 21%.[33]

Investigating Bone Perfusion in Osteoporosis

Recent evidence demonstrates the importance of bone perfusion in the health of bone[57–62] and that vascular dysfunction seen with aging is related to the pathogenesis of bone loss, osteoporosis, and fracture.[59,60,63–65] Bone perfusion is directly associated with the rate of bone remodeling activity.[66] However, to date perfusion in bone has been poorly studied, not least because most measurement techniques are difficult to apply in clinical studies.[58] It is possible to use ^{18}F-fluoride PET to estimate regional bone perfusion, and it has been applied successfully in several clinical studies.[21,22,29]

Van Dyke and colleagues[67] first proposed the use of ^{18}F-fluoride and a positron camera to quantify bone perfusion. Bone tracers enter the skeleton via osseous capillaries by diffusion, allowing bone perfusion to be estimated. The estimation is based on the assumption that the single-passage extraction efficiency of whole blood ^{18}F-fluoride by bone is 100%, which has been confirmed in an animal study by Wootton and Doré.[45] A highly significant correlation between bone perfusion estimated using ^{18}F-fluoride and true bone perfusion using the freely diffusible tracer ^{15}OH$_2$O has been reported using PET.[35,36]

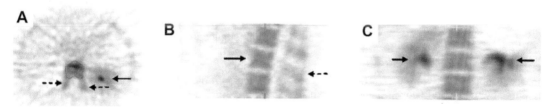

Fig. 3. (*A*) Transaxial ^{18}F-fluoride PET image of the lumbar vertebra showing the region of interest around the vertebral body (the *solid arrow* shows ^{18}F-fluoride activity within the kidney reflecting the normal excretory pathway of fluoride, and the *dashed arrows* show the posterior elements of the vertebral body including the pedicles). (*B*) Sagittal view (the *solid arrow* shows the vertebral body and the *dashed arrow* shows the spinous process). (*C*) Coronal view of ^{18}F-fluoride PET scan of lumbar spine (*solid arrows* show ^{18}F-fluoride activity within the kidneys). (*From* Frost ML, Blake GM, Cook GJ, et al. Differences in regional bone perfusion and turnover between lumbar spine and distal humerus: 18F-fluoride PET study of treatment-naïve and treated postmenopausal women. Bone 2009;45:942-8; with permission.)

However, this excellent agreement was only observed for low to moderate flow rates (≤ 0.16 mL min^{-1} mL^{-1}), with ^{18}F-fluoride PET progressively underestimating bone perfusion with increasing perfusion. The correlation was improved by correcting the ^{18}F-fluoride PET K_1 values for the permeability-surface area product of the tissue capillaries (**Fig. 4**). For ^{18}F-fluoride PET studies of healthy subjects and those with osteoporosis, it is likely that K_1 is a good approximation of bone perfusion because values of K_1 typically observed are significantly less than 0.16 mL min^{-1} mL^{-1}, even at metabolically active sites such as the lumbar spine.[22–24]

^{18}F-Fluoride PET studies have been performed to investigate differences in bone perfusion between skeletal sites. Highly significant variations have been observed between the lumbar spine and distal humerus.[21,26] In a study by Frost and colleagues,[26] 11 treatment-naïve postmenopausal women and 12 postmenopausal women on stable antiresorptive therapy had a dynamic PET scan of the lumbar spine and distal humerus after injection of 90 MBq ^{18}F-fluoride. Values of K_1 were on average 3 times greater at the lumbar spine compared with the humerus for both study groups.

This difference between skeletal sites was so pronounced that there was no overlap in the range of K_1 values observed at the spine (0.08–0.25 mL min^{-1} mL^{-1}) and humerus (0.01–0.07 mL min^{-1} mL^{-1}) for the treatment-naïve group (**Fig. 5**). A similar study was performed by the same research group on normal subjects, and revealed similar differences in bone perfusion between the lumbar spine and humerus.[21] Using a small rodent model and radiolabeled microspheres to measure blood flow, Bloomfield and colleagues[59] demonstrated significant variations in blood flow between skeletal sites for both adult and aged rats. These investigators also reported blood flow to the forelimb and femur to be almost 60% and 40% lower, respectively, in aged versus adult rats.[59] Diminishing bone perfusion with aging has also been observed in several other animal and clinical studies,[57,65,68] and reductions in blood flow have been observed in osteoporotic subjects compared with healthy controls.[65,69] As far as the authors are aware, an appropriately powered ^{18}F-fluoride PET study comparing bone perfusion in osteoporotic patients with normal subjects has not been reported. In a study comparing skeletal kinetics at the lumbar spine in postmenopausal women with and without osteoporosis, there was no significant difference in K_1 between groups (0.13 mL min^{-1} mL^{-1} vs 0.11 mL min^{-1} mL^{-1} for osteoporotic and normal subjects, respectively).[24] However, the precision error for K_1 is larger than that for K_i,[50] so the study was not adequately powered to detect significant differences in bone perfusion. Such a study is of importance, because reductions in bone perfusion are associated with greater bone loss[62] and there is a direct relationship between bone perfusion and bone remodeling activity.[32,66] ^{18}F-fluoride PET may also have a role in the measurement of bone perfusion following fracture or bone grafts to assess bone viability and predict the risk of necrosis.[27,70–74]

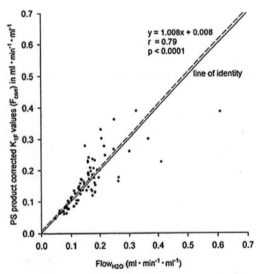

Fig. 4. Relationship between "true" arterial blood flow measured by ^{15}OH$_2$O PET (Flow$_{H2O}$) and permeability-surface product corrected regional blood flow estimates using ^{18}F-fluoride PET (F$_{corr}$) measured in porcine vertebrae. Linear regression analysis revealed a highly significant correlation between F$_{corr}$ and Flow$_{H2O}$ for the whole range of blood flow values (*dashed line*). (*Reprinted from* Piert M, Zittel TT, Machulla HJ, et al. Blood flow measurements with ^{15}OH$_2$O and ^{18}F-fluoride ion PET in porcine vertebrae. J Bone Miner Res 1998;13(8):1328–36; with permission.)

Examining Skeletal Heterogeneity

With significant differences between skeletal sites in age-related bone loss, disease progression and response to treatment it is more informative to examine regional rather than global differences in bone perfusion and bone turnover, particularly as it allows comparisons to be made between sites with varying amounts of trabecular and cortical bone. Despite cortical bone representing 80% of skeletal mass, the effects of aging, disease, or therapies, and its contribution to bone strength,[75] are often overlooked.[76] Using a rodent model and bone-seeking labels including tritiated tetracycline and ^{45}Ca, Cheong and colleagues[77]

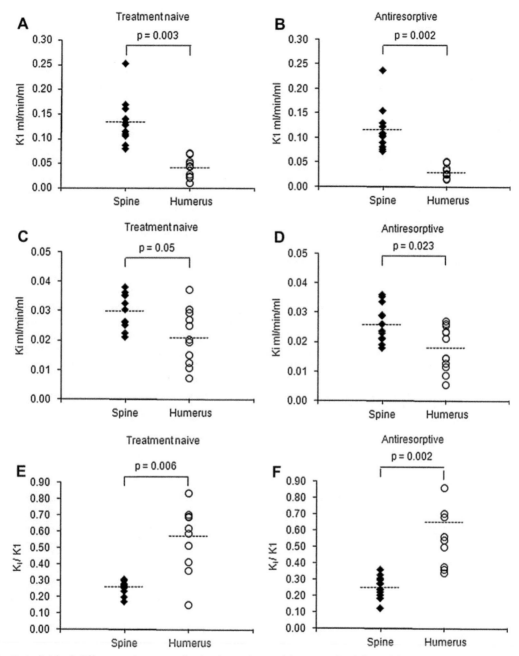

Fig. 5. Individual differences between the lumbar spine and humerus for (*A*) K_1, (*C*) K_i, and (*E*) K_i/K_1 for treatment-naïve postmenopausal women, and (*B*) K_1, (*D*) K_i, and (*F*) K_i/K_1 for postmenopausal women treated with antiresorptive drugs. The difference between skeletal sites was statistically significant for all parameters. (*Reprinted from* Frost ML, Blake GM, Cook GJ, et al. Differences in regional bone perfusion and turnover between lumbar spine and distal humerus: ^{18}F-fluoride PET study of treatment-naïve and treated postmenopausal women. Bone 2009;45(5):942–8; with permission.)

reported greater label incorporation at bone sites that were trabecular rich and therefore more metabolically active compared with skeletal sites consisting primarily of cortical bone such as the femoral mid-shaft. Differences between trabecular and cortical bone have been observed in response to aging,[78–81] microgravity,[82,83] and disease.[79,81,84] The rate of bone formation and the duration of each bone remodeling cycle has been shown to differ between cortical and trabecular bone,[85,86] as have the concentrations of bone-related proteins including osteocalcin and osteonectin.[87] Significant contributors to this variability in bone turnover between skeletal sites include differences in the surface to volume ratio, varying loading patterns, and the amount and characteristics of hematopoietic tissue.

Using quantitative bone SPECT, significant variations in bone turnover between the spine and femur have been reported in women with and without osteoporosis.[88,89] Although ^{18}F-fluoride PET provides information about bone at the regional level, very few articles have been published comparing bone turnover estimated using measurements of K_i, at different skeletal sites. Cook and colleagues[21] examined differences in skeletal kinetics between vertebral and humeral bone using dynamic ^{18}F-fluoride PET in 26 postmenopausal women without osteoporosis. The vertebral and humeral ROI time-activity curves were visually discrepant, with greater activity per unit volume within the vertebral bodies (**Fig. 6**). Plasma clearance of fluoride to bone mineral (K_i) and the unidirectional plasma clearance of fluoride to total bone tissue (K_1) were significantly greater at the lumbar spine compared with the humerus.[21] A similar study was performed by the same research group on patients with osteoporosis or significant

osteopenia, as described earlier.[26] In this study values of K_i were on average 50% greater at the lumbar spine compared with the humerus for both treatment-naïve subjects and those on antiresorptive therapy (see **Fig. 5**).[26] When fluoride kinetics was assessed in nonaffected bones in patients with Paget disease the highest values of K_i and SUV were observed at the vertebra, iliac bone, and scapula, and the lowest values were observed at the tibia and fibula.[29] These results emphasize that the rate of bone turnover estimated for the entire skeleton using biochemical markers or at one skeletal site by bone biopsy cannot be regarded as a generalized phenomenon, accurately reflecting bone turnover at all skeletal sites.

The ratio K_i/K_1 describing the unidirectional extraction efficiency to bone mineral was significantly greater at the humerus than at the lumbar spine for both study groups in the study by Frost and colleagues[26] (see **Fig. 5**), a finding also reported in the study by Cook and colleagues[21] of postmenopausal women with normal BMD. This result may reflect the greater access of fluoride to the bone mineral surface within the humeral extracellular fluid (ECF) space resulting from the smaller amount of marrow in a relatively cortical-rich site such as the distal humerus as compared with the lumbar spine.

Of particular interest in the osteoporosis field is the difference in bone turnover between the lumbar spine and hip. These skeletal sites are the 2 most common fracture sites associated with low BMD, and increases in BMD and reductions in fracture risk at these sites remain the primary outcomes of phase 3 therapeutic confirmatory trials of novel drugs for osteoporosis. Examining differences between sites in both bone metabolism and bone perfusion would allow a better understanding of the differential responses of treatment at different skeletal sites. As far as the authors are aware there have only been 2 studies, limited by the use of a static rather than dynamic scan protocols, which compared SUV at the lumbar spine and hip.[37,90] The study by Frost and colleagues[90] included postmenopausal women with osteoporosis or significant osteopenia. SUV at the lumbar spine (5.2 ± 1.0) were significantly greater than those at the femoral neck (2.7 ± 0.5, P<.001), femoral shaft (2.7 ± 0.6, P<.001), and entire proximal femur (2.6 ± 0.4, P<.001). The study by Uchida and colleagues[37] reported significantly lower SUV at the femoral neck than at the lumbar spine in women treated with corticosteroids. Further work is required, using dynamic PET scan protocols, to compare bone

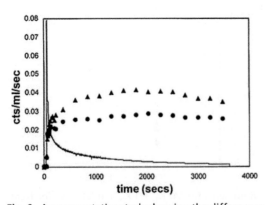

Fig. 6. A representative study showing the differences between the time-activity curves for lumbar vertebra (*triangles*) and humeral (*circles*) ROIs measured in postmenopausal women using ^{18}F-fluoride PET. An arterial plasma input function is also shown. The vertebral and humeral values have been multiplied by 5 for easier comparison with the input function. (*Reprinted from* Cook GJR, Lodge MA, Blake GM, et al. Differences in skeletal kinetics between vertebral and humeral bone measured by ^{18}F-fluoride positron emission tomography in postmenopausal women. J Bone Miner Res 2000;15:763–9; with permission.)

perfusion and bone turnover at the spine and hip, in particular in response to treatment.

Assessment of Fracture Healing

Relatively little basic or clinical research has been performed to investigate whether fracture healing is altered in patients with osteoporosis.[91] To date, reports have been conflicting and limited by the imaging modalities used for the assessment of the fracture healing process. An improved understanding of the healing process combined with an ability to assess the effects of surgical or therapeutic interventions that have the potential to reduce the risk of nonunion or accelerate fracture healing would be beneficial. Further, it has been shown that drugs initially developed for the treatment of osteoporosis may also positively influence fracture healing and implant fixation following orthopedic surgery.[92] The use of ^{18}F-fluoride PET for the evaluation of fracture healing is attractive as, unlike other imaging modalities, it can provide quantitative information on bone perfusion and

turnover, and may allow the early prediction of delayed fracture healing, nonunion of long bone fractures,[93] or joint implant failure. Hsu and colleagues[93] used a rat femur model to assess fracture healing in a sophisticated study using ^{18}F-fluoride and ^{18}F-FDG PET. Animals underwent either standard femoral fractures using a 3-point bending technique (Group I) or osteotomy and insertion of a 22-mm silastic spacer (Group 2), to represent a standard fracture and nonunion, respectively. Plain radiographs and static PET scans were performed at 1, 2, 3, and 4 weeks post fracture. ROI were drawn on coronal view encompassing the fracture site and SUV calculated. Histologic analysis was performed following euthanasia. Uptake of ^{18}F-fluoride was significantly greater at all time points for Group 1 compared with Group 2, and SUV increased with time post fracture in Group 1, demonstrating that increased bone formation was associated with fracture healing. In contrast, ^{18}F-FDG uptake was not significantly different between groups and did not change with time in Group 1. **Fig. 7** shows the plain radiographs and

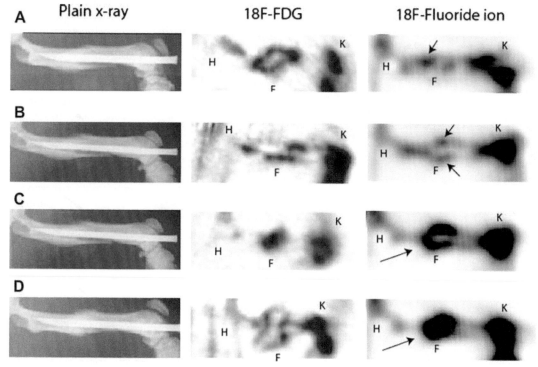

Fig. 7. Plain radiographs and corresponding ^{18}F-FDG and ^{18}F-fluoride PET images of a rat femur following femoral fracture at 1 week (*A*), 2 weeks (*B*), 3 weeks (*C*), and 4 weeks (*D*) post fracture. Subjective evaluation of plain radiographs of the femur did not show any discernible callus formation until 2 weeks post fracture. ^{18}F-fluoride images show increased uptake in the fracture union site during fracture repair at all time points (*arrows*). By contrast, no significant differences were seen in ^{18}F-FDG tracer uptake at any time point. K, knee; F, fracture site; H, hip. (*Reprinted from* Hsu WK, Feeley BT, Krenek L, et al. The use of ^{18}F-fluoride and ^{18}F-FDG PET scans to assess fracture healing in a rat femur model. Eur J Nucl Med Mol Imaging 2007;34(8):1291–301; with permission.)

corresponding ^{18}F-FDG and ^{18}F-fluoride PET images for each time point for Group 1. **Fig. 8** shows the images for animals from Group 2, highlighting minimal uptake (SUV <1 at all time points) at the fracture site and subsequently poor fracture healing potential, thus illustrating how the PET images provide more obvious differences between time points compared with the subtle variations seen on radiographs.[93] Therefore, such images could have a role in the assessment of longitudinal fracture healing that may be superior to subjective assessment of radiographs by orthopedic surgeons, and may also help predict the development of nonunion earlier than conventional methods. Silva and colleagues[94] reported increased fluoride uptake with fatigue loading in the forelimb of adult rats, indicating that ^{18}F-fluoride PET may also have a role in quantifying the magnitude of the skeletal response to stress fractures, commonly seen in the lower extremities in athletes and military recruits. Further research is required to determine the efficacy of ^{18}F-fluoride in clinical practice for these indications.

Evaluation of Novel Drugs for Osteoporosis

Potentially the most exciting and clinically useful role of ^{18}F-fluoride PET is the evaluation of novel drugs being developed for the treatment of osteoporosis and other metabolic bone diseases. Conventional methods do not allow an assessment of the direct effects of drugs on bone turnover at clinically important sites such as the lumbar spine and hip. Further significant changes in bone density in response to treatment can take many months and even several years to detect, even at the most favorable measurement site such as the lumbar spine.[95] Biochemical markers of bone turnover, a global measure of skeletal function, are typically used as surrogate end points in early-phase clinical trials. However, a knowledge of the direct effects of a drug on regional bone turnover at common osteoporotic fractures sites, which could be observed over a relatively short time period (ie, weeks rather than months or years) would be invaluable and may aid in the "go/no-go" decision when

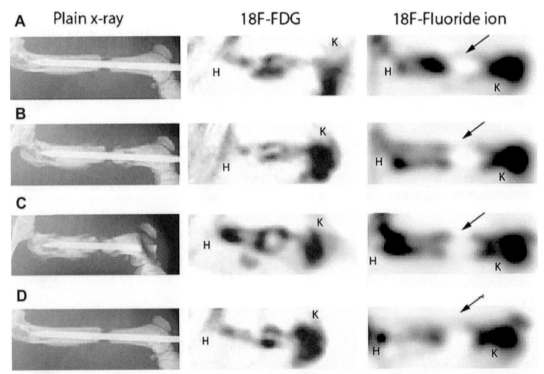

Fig. 8. Plain radiographs and corresponding ^{18}F-FDG and ^{18}F-fluoride PET images of a rat femur following femoral fracture and insertion of 2 mm silastic spacer to represent nonunion of fracture at 1 week (*A*), 2 weeks (*B*), 3 weeks (*C*), and 4 weeks (*D*) post fracture. ^{18}F-fluoride PET images show tracer uptake extending into fracture site from the bony ends (*arrows*); however, uptake is minimal (SUV <1 at all time points), indicating poor fracture healing potential. Significant localized uptake of ^{18}F-FDG is seen at all time points despite absence of bone formation at fracture site. This preclinical study supports the plausibility of using ^{18}F-fluoride PET imaging to evaluate fracture healing and risk of nonunion. K, knee; H, hip. (*Reprinted from* Hsu WK, Feeley BT, Krenek L, et al. The use of ^{18}F-fluoride and ^{18}F-FDG PET scans to assess fracture healing in a rat femur model. Eur J Nucl Med Mol Imaging 2007;34(8):1291–301; with permission.)

considering which drugs should be assessed further in pivotal phase 3 fracture outcome trials. For example, a drug that is shown to have a potent effect on bone turnover at the proximal femur using ^{18}F-fluoride PET could then be advanced for later phase development.

In a study of 18 women with osteoporosis or significant osteopenia treated with risedronate, an antiresorptive agent, K_i measured at the lumbar spine using ^{18}F-fluoride PET was significantly decreased by 18% following 6 months of treatment.[23] This decrease in K_i was similar in magnitude to that observed in biochemical markers of bone turnover measured in the same subjects at the same time points. This study was the first to demonstrate the direct metabolic effect of an anti-resorptive therapy on skeletal kinetics at the lumbar spine in patients with osteoporosis.[23] Uchida and colleagues[37] used ^{18}F-fluoride PET to examine longitudinal changes in bone remodeling with alendronate treatment in patients on 10 mg or more glucocorticoids. Lumbar spine and femoral neck SUV levels significantly decreased following 3 and 12 months of alendronate treatment. Global markers of bone turnover also decreased significantly and, as expected, there was a significant improvement in both spine and hip BMD.[37] In a 6-month prospective study of 14 patients with monostotic or polyostotic Paget disease treated with bisphosphonates, K_i decreased significantly within 1 month of therapy by approximately 28% and a further decrease of approximately 24% was observed at 6 months.[29] In the same study the correlation between K_i using nonlinear regression, K_i calculated using Patlak analysis, and SUV max were highly correlated at baseline as were the changes observed in each parameter over time.[29] Further research is required to fully investigate the potential of ^{18}F-fluoride PET as a tool for assessing the efficacy of novel drugs on regional bone turnover. Studies should include direct comparison with conventional methods, including the gold standard of bone biopsy, and an assessment of the sensitivity of the different parameters of interest using different analytical methodologies for detecting response to treatment.

Assessment of Other Metabolic Bone Diseases

In addition to patients with osteoporosis, ^{18}F-fluoride PET has also been used to examine bone perfusion and bone turnover in patients with Paget disease and renal osteodystrophy. Paget disease is a benign bone disorder characterized by increased bone formation and bone resorption. Paget disease can affect single (monostotic) or several skeletal sites (polyostotic), so global biochemical markers can be normal in patients with monostotic disease and may not accurately represent disease activity with polyostotic disease. ^{18}F-Fluoride PET may be of value in focal diseases such as Paget, as it allows the direct assessment of bone perfusion and turnover in the pagetic bone that can then be compared with either nonaffected bone in the same patient (as long as a normal contralateral bone is within the field of view) or with normal reported values if available. In a study of 14 patients with Paget disease, values of K_i and SUV, assessed at several skeletal sites, were significantly greater in pagetic than in normal bone.[29] The mean ratio of pagetic to normal bone was 5.91 for SUV_{max}, 7.32 for K_i derived using Patlak analysis, and 7.25 for K_i derived using nonlinear regression.[29] Cook and colleagues[22] compared dynamic ^{18}F-fluoride PET parameters in vertebral pagetic bone with normal bone. Seven pagetic patients with known vertebral involvement using bone scintigraphy underwent a dynamic ^{18}F-fluoride PET scan of the lumbar spine. Qualitative assessment of the PET images clearly showed increased uptake of fluoride compared with adjacent nonaffected vertebrae (**Fig. 9**). Values of plasma clearance to total bone

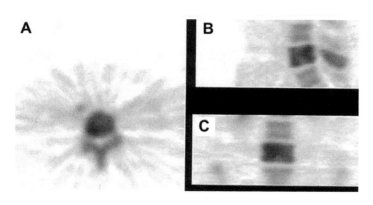

A   **B**   **C**

Fig. 9. ^{18}F-fluoride PET image of the lumbar spine showing increased uptake of tracer in a pagetic lumbar vertebra. (A) Transaxial; (B) sagittal; (C) coronal. (*Reprinted from* Cook GJR, Blake GM, Marsden PK, et al. Quantification of skeletal kinetic indices in Paget's disease using dynamic ^{18}F-fluoride positron emission tomography. J Bone Miner Res 2002;17:854–9; with permission.)

tissue (K_1) and bone mineral (K_i) were on average 3 and 2 times greater, respectively, in pagetic vertebra compared with normal bone.[22]

Mineral homeostasis becomes increasingly compromised in patients with chronic renal disease, leading to a variety of bone disorders characterized by abnormal bone turnover, coupling, and mineralization.[96] Renal osteodystrophy (ROD) represents a spectrum of skeletal disorders ranging from reduced bone turnover and/or impaired mineralization, such as that seen with adynamic bone disease and osteomalacia, to high-turnover disorders such as hyperparathyroidism and osteitis fibrosa.[97] As with osteoporosis, bone biopsy remains the gold standard for diagnosing the major categories of renal bone disease.[18,96] The major disadvantages of its invasive nature, complexity, and cost has led to the use of biochemical markers, in particular parathyroid hormone (PTH), as an alternative method for diagnosing bone turnover abnormalities.[18] Assays for PTH have been widely used over the past 2 decades for classifying, monitoring, and treating ROD. However, PTH levels do not always agree with data obtained from histologic studies.[18] ^{18}F-fluoride PET may have a role in quantifying bone turnover in patients with ROD, in particular in classifying patients with the 2 extremes of bone turnover, specifically adynamic bone disease and hyperparathyroidism. This assessment would be especially useful for the diagnosis of adynamic bone disease, which although common cannot be readily diagnosed in clinical practice other than by bone biopsy, which is rarely performed. In a relatively small study of 11 patients with renal osteodystrophy, Messa and colleagues[31] demonstrated that the plasma clearance of fluoride to bone mineral was significantly higher in patients with secondary hyperparathyroidism than in normal subjects and in patients with adynamic bone disease. Of note, they also reported highly significant correlations between K_i and histomorphometric indices of bone formation rate ($r = 0.84$, $P<.01$). Clinical studies are required to assess the sensitivity and specificity of ^{18}F-fluoride PET in detecting bone turnover abnormalities in patients with renal osteodystrophy as compared with intact PTH measurements to determine whether the former is superior to the latter, which has the major advantages of being cheap and simple to perform but may lack sensitivity.

SUMMARY AND FURTHER WORK

Although complex and relatively costly, ^{18}F-fluoride PET offers important advantages over conventional methods for quantifying the rate of bone turnover activity. In addition, it allows the simultaneous assessment of bone perfusion, the importance of which is increasingly being recognized in osteoporosis. Because of the complexity of scan acquisition and analysis protocols associated with dynamic scanning, it would be attractive to estimate bone turnover using the SUV index, widely used for clinical FDG studies. However, the accuracy of SUV as an estimate of bone turnover has not yet been assessed. Further dynamic PET has only been directly compared with the gold standard of bone biopsy and histomorphometric analysis in 2 sophisticated but small studies, so a large clinical study is essential. ^{18}F-Fluoride PET now has an established role as a research technique, and there is clearly a need for further studies to fully examine the potential role of ^{18}F-fluoride PET in the assessment of the pathophysiology of osteoporosis and the evaluation of novel pharmaceutical treatments for this and other metabolic bone disorders.

REFERENCES

1. Consensus development conference: diagnosis prophylaxis and treatment of osteoporosis. Am J Med 1993;94:646–50.
2. Boonen S, Singer AJ. Osteoporosis management: impact of fracture type on cost and quality of life in patients at risk for fracture I. Curr Med Res Opin 2008;24(6):1781–8.
3. Department of Health. Advisory Group on Osteoporosis. London: Department of Health; 1994.
4. Cole ZA, Dennison EM, Cooper C. Osteoporosis epidemiology update. Curr Rheumatol Rep 2008; 10(2):92–6.
5. Johnell O, Kanis JA, Oden A, et al. Predictive value of BMD for hip and other fractures. J Bone Miner Res 2005;20(7):1185–94.
6. World Health Organization (WHO). Assessment of fracture risk and its application to screening for postmenopausal osteoporosis. Report of a WHO Study Group. World Health Organ Tech Rep Ser 1994;843:1–129, World Health Organization, Geneva, Switzerland.
7. Cranney A, Jamal SA, Tsang JF, et al. Low bone mineral density and fracture burden in postmenopausal women. CMAJ 2007;177(6):575–80.
8. Kanis JA, Oden A, Johnell O, et al. The use of clinical risk factors enhances the performance of BMD in the prediction of hip and osteoporotic fractures in men and women. Osteoporos Int 2007;18(8): 1033–46.
9. Kanis JA, Johnell O, Oden A, et al. FRAX and the assessment of fracture probability in men and women from the UK. Osteoporos Int 2008;19(4):385–97.

10. Kanis JA, McCloskey EV, Johansson H, et al. Case finding for the management of osteoporosis with FRAX-assessment and intervention thresholds for the UK. Osteoporos Int 2008;19(10): 1395–408.

11. Heaney RP. Is the paradigm shifting? Bone 2003;33: 457–65.

12. Kleerekoper M. Overview of osteoporosis treatment. In: Rosen CJ, Compston JE, Lian JB, editors. Primer on the metabolic bone diseases and disorders of mineral metabolism. 7th edition. Washington, DC: American Society of Bone and Mineral Research; 2008. p. 220–1.

13. Garnero P, Sornay-Rendu E, Duboef F, et al. Markers of bone turnover for the prediction of fracture risk. Osteoporos Int 1999;11(Suppl 6):55–65.

14. Johnell O, Oden A, De Laet C, et al. Biochemical indices of bone turnover and the assessment of fracture probability. Osteoporos Int 2002;13:523–6.

15. Eastell R, Barton I, Hannon RA. Relationship of early changes in bone resorption to the reduction in fracture risk with risedronate. J Bone Miner Res 2003;18: 1051–6.

16. Hochberg MC, Greenspan S, Wasnich RD, et al. Changes in bone density and turnover explain the reduction in incidence of nonvertebral fractures that occur during treatment with antiresorptive agents. J Clin Endocrinol Metab 2002;87:1586–92.

17. Compston JE, Croucher PI. Histomorphometric assessment of trabecular bone remodelling in osteoporosis. Bone Miner 1991;14:91–102.

18. Martin KJ, Olgaard K, on behalf of the Bone Turnover Work Group. Diagnosis, assessment, and treatment of bone turnover abnormalities in renal osteodystrophy. Am J Kidney Dis 2004;43:558–65.

19. Delmas PD, Eastell R, Garnero P, et al. for the Committee of Scientific Advisors of the International Osteoporosis Foundation. The use of biochemical markers of bone turnover in osteoporosis. Osteoporos Int 2000;11(Suppl 6):2–17.

20. Seibel MJ. Molecular markers of bone turnover: biochemical, technical and analytical aspects. Osteoporos Int 2000;11(Suppl 6):18–29.

21. Cook GJ, Lodge MA, Blake GM, et al. Differences in skeletal kinetics between vertebral and humeral bone measured by 18F-fluoride positron emission tomography in postmenopausal women. J Bone Miner Res 2000;15:763–9.

22. Cook GJR, Blake GM, Marsden PK, et al. Quantification of skeletal kinetic indices in Paget's disease using dynamic 18F-fluoride positron emission tomography. J Bone Miner Res 2002;17:854–9.

23. Frost ML, Cook GJR, Blake GM, et al. A prospective study of risedronate on regional bone metabolism and blood flow at the lumbar spine measured by 18F-fluoride positron emission tomography. J Bone Miner Res 2003;18:2215–22.

24. Frost ML, Cook GJR, Blake GM, et al. Dissociation between global markers of bone formation and direct measurement of spinal bone formation in osteoporosis. J Bone Miner Res 2004; 19:1797–804.

25. Frost ML, Cook GJR, Blake GM, et al. The relationship between regional bone turnover measured using 18F-fluoride positron emission tomography and changes in BMD is equivalent to that seen for biochemical markers of bone turnover. J Clin Densitom 2006;10:46–54.

26. Frost ML, Blake GM, Cook GJ, et al. Differences in regional bone perfusion and turnover between lumbar spine and distal humerus: 18F-fluoride PET study of treatment-naïve and treated postmenopausal women. Bone 2009;45(5):942–8.

27. Brenner W, Vernon C, Muzi M, et al. Comparison of different quantitative approaches to 18F-fluoride PET scans. J Nucl Med 2004;45:1493–500.

28. Hawkins RA, Choi Y, Huang S-C, et al. Evaluation of the skeletal kinetics of fluorine-18-fluoride ion with PET. J Nucl Med 1992;33:633–42.

29. Installe J, Nzeusseu A, Bol A, et al. 18F-fluoride PET for monitoring therapeutic response in Paget's disease of bone. J Nucl Med 2005;46:1650–8.

30. Moore AE, Blake GM, Taylor KA, et al. Assessment of regional changes in skeletal metabolism following 3 and 18 months of teriparatide treatment. J Bone Miner Res 2009. [Epub ahead of print].

31. Messa C, Goodman WG, Hoh CK, et al. Bone metabolic activity measured with positron emission tomography and 18F-fluoride ion in renal osteodystrophy: correlation with bone histomorphometry. J Clin Endocrinol Metab 1993;77:949–55.

32. Piert M, Zittel TT, Becker GA, et al. Assessment of porcine bone metabolism by dynamic 18F-fluoride PET: correlation with bone histomorphometry. J Nucl Med 2001;42:1091–100.

33. Piert M, Zittel TT, Jahn M, et al. Increased sensitivity in detection of a porcine high-turnover osteopenia after total gastrectomy by dynamic 18F-fluoride ion PET and quantitative CT. J Nucl Med 2003;44: 117–24.

34. Schiepers C, Nuyts J, Bormans G, et al. Fluoride kinetics of the axial skeleton measured in vivo with fluorine-18-fluoride PET. J Nucl Med 1997; 38:1970–6.

35. Piert M, Zittel TT, Machulla HJ, et al. Blood flow measurements with 15OH2O and 18F-fluoride ion PET in porcine vertebrae. J Bone Miner Res 1998; 13(8):1328–36.

36. Piert M, Machulla H-J, Jahn M, et al. Coupling of porcine bone blood flow and metabolism in high-turnover bone disease measured by 15OH2O and 18F-fluoride ion positron emission tomography. Eur J Nucl Med 2002;29:907–14.

37. Uchida K, Nakajima H, Miyazaki T, et al. Effects of alendronate on bone metabolism in glucocorticoid-induced osteoporosis measured by ^{18}F-fluoride PET: a prospective study. J Nucl Med 2009;50(11):1808–14.

38. Berding G, Kirchhoff TD, Burchert W, et al. ^{18}F-fluoride PET indicates reduced bone formation in severe glucocorticoid-induced osteoporosis. Nuklearmedizin 1998;37(2):76–9.

39. Blau M, Nagler W, Bender MA. Fluorine-18: a new isotope for bone scanning. J Nucl Med 1962;3:332–4.

40. Ishiguro K, Nakagaki H, Tsuboi S, et al. Distribution of fluoride in cortical bone of human rib. Calcif Tissue Int 1993;52:278–82.

41. Narita N, Kato K, Nakagaki H, et al. Distribution of fluoride concentration in the rat's bone. Calcif Tissue Int 1990;46:200–4.

42. Grant FD, Fahey FH, Packard AB, et al. Skeletal PET with ^{18}F-fluoride: applying new technology to an old tracer. J Nucl Med 2008;49(1):68–78.

43. Blake GM, Park-Holohan SJ, Cook GJ, et al. Quantitative studies of bone with the use of ^{18}F-fluoride and ^{99m}Tc-methylene diphosphonate. Semin Nucl Med 2001;31(1):28–49.

44. Hosking DJ, Chamberlain MJ. Studies in man with 18F. Clin Sci 1972;42(2):153–61.

45. Wootton R, Doré C. The single-passage extraction of ^{18}F in rabbit bone. Clin Phys Physiol Meas 1986;7(4):333–43.

46. Schirrmeister H, Guhlmann A, Elsner K, et al. Sensitivity in detecting osseous lesions depends on anatomic localization: planar bone scintigraphy versus ^{18}F PET. J Nucl Med 1999;40(10):1623–9.

47. Schirrmeister H, Glatting G, Hetzel J, et al. Prospective evaluation of the clinical value of planar bone scans, SPECT, and (18)F-labeled NaF PET in newly diagnosed lung cancer. J Nucl Med 2001;42(12):1800–4.

48. Hetzel M, Arslandemir C, König HH, et al. F-18 NaF PET for detection of bone metastases in lung cancer: accuracy, cost-effectiveness, and impact on patient management. J Bone Miner Res 2003;18(12):2206–14.

49. Even-Sapir E, Metser U, Flusser G, et al. Assessment of malignant skeletal disease: initial experience with ^{18}F-fluoride PET/CT and comparison between ^{18}F-fluoride PET and ^{18}F-fluoride PET/CT. J Nucl Med 2004;45(2):272–8.

50. Frost ML, Blake GM, Park-Holohan SJ, et al. Long-term precision of ^{18}F-fluoride PET skeletal kinetic studies in the assessment of bone metabolism. J Nucl Med 2008;49:700–7.

51. Arlot ME, Delmas PD, Chappard D, et al. Trabecular and endocortical bone remodelling in postmenopausal osteoporosis: comparison with normal postmenopausal women. Osteoporos Int 1990;1:41–9.

52. Eriksen EF, Hodgson SF, Eastell R, et al. Cancellous bone remodelling in type I (postmenopausal) osteoporosis: quantitative assessment of rates of formation, resorption, and bone loss at tissue and cellular levels. J Bone Miner Res 1990;5:311–9.

53. Garcia-Carasco M, de Vernejoul MC, Sterkers Y, et al. Decreased bone formation in osteoporotic patients compared with age-matched controls. Calcif Tissue Int 1989;44:173–5.

54. Kimmel DB, Recker RR, Gallagher JC, et al. A comparison of iliac bone histomorphometric data in postmenopausal osteoporotic and normal subjects. Bone Miner 1990;11:217–35.

55. Parfitt AM, Villanueva AR, Foldes J, et al. Relations between histologic indices of bone formation: implications for the pathogenesis of spinal osteoporosis. J Bone Miner Res 1995;10:466–73.

56. Canalis E, Delany AM. Mechanisms of glucocorticoid action in bone. Ann N Y Acad Sci 2002;966:73–81.

57. Prisby RD, Ramsey MW, Behnke BJ, et al. Aging reduces skeletal blood flow, endothelium-dependent vasodilation, and NO bioavailability in rats. J Bone Miner Res 2007;22:1280–8.

58. McCarthy I. The physiology of bone blood flow: a review. J Bone Joint Surg Am 2006;88(Suppl 3):4–9.

59. Bloomfield SA, Hogan HA, Delp MD. Decreases in bone blood flow and bone material properties in aging Fischer-344 rats. Clin Orthop Relat Res 2002;396:248–57.

60. Griffith JF, Yeung DK, Tsang PH, et al. Compromised bone marrow perfusion in osteoporosis. J Bone Miner Res 2008;23:1068–75.

61. Eriksen EF, Eghbali-Fatourechi GZ, Khosla S. Remodeling and vascular spaces in bone. J Bone Miner Res 2007;22:1–6.

62. Vogt MT, Cauley JA, Kuller LH, et al. Bone mineral density and blood flow to the lower extremities: the study of osteoporotic fractures. J Bone Miner Res 1997;12:283–9.

63. Alagiakrishnan K, Juby A, Hanley D, et al. Role of vascular factors in osteoporosis. J Gerontol A Biol Sci Med Sci 2003;58:362–6.

64. Sanada M, Taguchi A, Higashi Y, et al. Forearm endothelial function and bone mineral loss in postmenopausal women. Atherosclerosis 2004;176:387–92.

65. Laroche M, Ludot I, Thiechart M, et al. Study of the intraosseous vessels of the femoral head in patients with fractures of the femoral neck or osteoarthritis of the hip. Osteoporos Int 1995;5:213–7.

66. Reeve J, Arlot M, Wootton R, et al. Skeletal blood flow, iliac histomorphometry, and strontium kinetics in osteoporosis: a relationship between blood flow and corrected apposition rate. J Clin Endocrinol Metab 1988;66:1124–31.

67. Van Dyke D, Anger HO, Yano Y, et al. Bone blood flow shown with F18 and the positron camera. Am J Physiol 1965;209:65–70.

68. Shih TT, Liu HC, Chang CJ, et al. Correlation of MR lumbar spine bone marrow perfusion with bone mineral density in female subjects. Radiology 2004;233(1):121–8.

69. Griffith JF, Yeung DK, Antonio GE, et al. Vertebral marrow fat content and diffusion and perfusion indexes in women with varying bone density: MR evaluation. Radiology 2006;241:831–8.

70. Schiepers C, Broos P, Miserez M, et al. Measurement of skeletal flow with positron emission tomography and 18F-fluoride in femoral head osteonecrosis. Arch Orthop Trauma Surg 1998;118(3):131–5.

71. Ullmark G, Sörensen J, Långström B, et al. Bone regeneration 6 years after impaction bone grafting: a PET analysis. Acta Orthop 2007;78(2):201–5.

72. Schliephake H, Berding G, Knapp WH, et al. Monitoring of graft perfusion and osteoblast activity in revascularised fibula segments using [18F]-positron emission tomography. Int J Oral Maxillofac Surg 1999;28(5):349–55.

73. Piert M, Winter E, Becker GA, et al. Allogenic bone graft viability after hip revision arthroplasty assessed by dynamic [18F]fluoride ion positron emission tomography. Eur J Nucl Med 1999;26(6):615–24.

74. Temmerman OP, Raijmakers PG, Heyligers IC, et al. Bone metabolism after total hip revision surgery with impacted grafting: evaluation using H2 15O and [18F]fluoride PET; a pilot study. Mol Imaging Biol 2008;10(5):288–93.

75. Andresen R, Werner HJ, Schober HC. Contribution of the cortical shell of vertebrae to mechanical behaviour of the lumbar vertebrae with implications for predicting fracture risk. Br J Radiol 1998;71:759–65.

76. Rico H. The therapy of osteoporosis and the importance of cortical bone. Calcif Tissue Int 1997;61:431–2.

77. Cheong JM, Gunaratna NS, McCabe GP, et al. Bone seeking labels as markers for bone turnover: effect of dosing schedule on labeling various bone sites in rats. Calcif Tissue Int 2009;85:440–50.

78. Riggs BL, Melton LJ, Robb RA, et al. A population-based assessment of rates of bone loss at multiple skeletal sites: evidence for substantial trabecular bone loss in young adult women and men. J Bone Miner Res 2008;23:205–14.

79. Tsurusaki K, Ito M, Hayashi K. Differential effects of menopause and metabolic disease on trabecular and cortical bone assessed by peripheral quantitative computed tomography (pQCT). Br J Radiol 2000;73:14–22.

80. Meier DE, Orwoll ES, Jones JM. Marked disparity between trabecular and cortical bone loss with age in healthy men. Measurement by vertebral computed tomography and radial photon absorptiometry. Ann Intern Med 1984;101:605–12.

81. Rüegsegger P, Durand EP, Dambacher MA. Differential effects of aging and disease on trabecular and compact bone density of the radius. Bone 1991;12:99–105.

82. Vico L, Collet P, Guignandon A, et al. Effects of long-term microgravity exposure on cancellous and cortical weight-bearing bones of cosmonauts. Lancet 2000;355:1607–11.

83. Turner CH. Site-specific skeletal effects of exercise: importance of interstitial fluid pressure. Bone 1999;24:161–2.

84. Byers RJ, Denton J, Hoyland JA, et al. Differential patterns of altered bone formation in different bone compartments in established osteoporosis. J Clin Pathol 1999;52:23–8.

85. Eventov I, Frisch B, Cohen Z, et al. Osteopenia, hematopoiesis, and bone remodelling in iliac crest and femoral biopsies: a prospective study of 102 cases of femoral neck fractures. Bone 1991;12:1–6.

86. Pødenphant J, Engel U. Regional variations in histomorphometric bone dynamics from the skeleton of an osteoporotic woman. Calcif Tissue Int 1987;40:184–8.

87. Ninomiya JT, Tracy RP, Calore JD, et al. Heterogeneity of human bone. J Bone Miner Res 1990;5:933–8.

88. Carnevale V, Dicembrino F, Frusciante V, et al. Different patterns of global and regional skeletal uptake of 99mTc-methylene diphosphonate with age: relevance to the pathogenesis of bone loss. J Nucl Med 2000;41:1478–83.

89. Israel O, Lubushitzky R, Frenkel A, et al. Bone turnover in cortical and trabecular bone in normal women and in women with osteoporosis. J Nucl Med 1994;35:1155–8.

90. Frost ML, Cook GJR, Blake GM, et al. A comparison of regional bone turnover at the spine and hip in postmenopausal women with osteoporosis. Osteoporos Int 2004;15(Suppl 2):40–1.

91. Giannoudis P, Tzioupis C, Almalki T, et al. Fracture healing in osteoporotic fractures: is it really different? A basic science perspective. Injury 2007;38(Suppl 1):S90–9.

92. Barnes GL, Kakar S, Vora S, et al. Stimulation of fracture-healing with systemic intermittent parathyroid hormone treatment. J Bone Joint Surg Am 2008;90(Suppl 1):120–7.

93. Hsu WK, Feeley BT, Krenek L, et al. The use of 18F-fluoride and 18F-FDG PET scans to assess fracture healing in a rat femur model. Eur J Nucl Med Mol Imaging 2007;34(8):1291–301.

94. Silva MJ, Uthgenannt BA, Rutlin JR, et al. In vivo skeletal imaging of 18F-fluoride with positron emission tomography reveals damage- and time-dependent responses to fatigue loading in the rat ulna. Bone 2006;39(2):229–36.

95. Blake GM, Frost ML, Fogelman I. Quantitative radio-nuclide studies of bone. J Nucl Med 2009;50(11): 1747–50.

96. Elder G. Pathophysiology and recent advances in the management of renal osteodystrophy. J Bone Miner Res 2002;17:2094–105.

97. Goodman WG, Coburn JW, Slatopolsky E, et al. Renal osteodystrophy in adults and children. In: Favus MJ, editor. Primer on the metabolic bone diseases and disorders of mineral metabolism. 4th edition. Philadelphia: Lippincott Williams & Wilkins; 1999. p. 347–63.

18F-Fluoride PET and PET/CT Imaging of Skeletal Metastases

Gary J.R. Cook, MSc, MD, FRCR, FRCP

KEYWORDS

- 18F-fluoride • Positron emission tomography
- Skeletal metastases

Many cancers metastasize to the skeleton. For example, 70% of patients suffering from 2 of the commonest cancers, namely breast and prostate cancers, have evidence of skeletal involvement at post mortem.[1] Skeletal metastases are associated with significant morbidities, including pain, pathologic fracture, spinal cord compression, hypercalcemia, and bone marrow suppression. Although the presence of bone metastases is a poor prognostic feature in most cancers, in breast and prostate cancers the survival may be long (eg, 24 and 20 months median survival, respectively),[2] and metastatic skeletal disease therefore makes a significant effect on health care resources.

The diagnosis and follow-up of patients with skeletal metastases is therefore crucially important for their clinical management, and imaging techniques have traditionally played a major role in the evaluation of the skeleton. Historically, conventional bone scintigraphy, using 99mTc-labeled diphosphonates, has been most commonly used, but in recent years, improvements and development of other modalities including multidetector computed tomography (CT), magnetic resonance imaging (MRI), and PET have led to their greater use.

Although the 99mTc-labeled diphosphonates remain the most commonly used agents for functional skeletal assessment, the positron-emitting agent 18F sodium fluoride (18F-fluoride) was first described in 1962 (**Fig. 1**).[3] However, it was not until the development of clinical PET scanners in the 1990s and subsequently PET/CT scanners in the 2000s, with resultant improvement in image quality, that there has been a renewal of interest in using 18F-fluoride for assessing benign and malignant skeletal disease (**Fig. 2**).

MECHANISMS

It has been assumed that the skeletal clearance of 18F-fluoride ion is similar to the diphosphonates in that it depends on a combination of local blood flow and osteoblastic activity.[4] In vitro experiments have suggested that the uptake of this tracer is not dependent on osteoblast numbers but depends on the concentration of bone-forming minerals.[5] Confirmation that the uptake of 18F-fluoride preferentially reflects bone formation and mineralization is provided by Messa and colleagues'[6] work on subjects with renal osteodystrophy. Correlations have been shown in the spine between parameters reflecting plasma clearance of 18F-fluoride to bone mineral (K_i or K_{bone}) and other biochemical and histomorphometric markers and indices of bone formation. Evidence suggests that 18F-fluoride undergoes high first-pass extraction approaching 100% in bone at physiologic blood flow rates, therefore allowing the estimation of bone blood flow (K_1 or K_{total}).[7] There is subsequent chemisorption into bone crystals, with the formation of fluoroapatite, and this process occurs preferentially at sites of actively mineralizing bone.[8,9] Once 18F-fluoride is incorporated onto the bone crystal surface, it is essentially trapped and only released when the bone is remodeled. Unlike diphosphonates, 18F-fluoride is not protein

Department of Nuclear Medicine and PET, The Royal Marsden NHS Foundation Trust, Downs Road, Sutton SM2 5PT, UK
E-mail address: gcook@icr.ac.uk

PET Clin 5 (2010) 275–280
doi:10.1016/j.cpet.2010.02.006

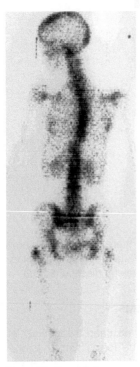

Fig. 1. A rectilinear ^{18}F-fluoride bone scan of a patient with metastatic breast cancer performed in 1973 in Guys Hospital, London.

bound, and because skeletal uptake is rapid, it is possible to obtain scans as soon as 1 hour after injection.[10] Another difference between ^{18}F-fluoride and ^{99m}Tc diphosphonates is that the former undergoes some renal tubular reabsorption after filtration that is sensitive to urine flow rate, whereas the latter is excreted after filtration.[4] High lesion-to-background ratios are obtained with ^{18}F-fluoride at 1 hour at sites of metastatic disease in both osteoblastic and osteolytic metastases, with metastatic sites showing a 5 to 10 times higher transport rate constant for ^{18}F-fluoride trapping compared with normal bone.[11] An injected activity of 250 MBq allows high-quality skeletal images on modern PET imaging systems, with a radiation dose of approximately 6 mSv to the patient.[12]

Semiquantitative measurements of ^{18}F-fluoride uptake are possible with static PET acquisitions; it is also possible to measure regional kinetic parameters from dynamic PET acquisitions if the arterial input function is also measured.[13] A 3-compartment model was first described by Hawkins, including plasma, bone extracellular fluid, and bone mineral compartments.[14] It is possible to estimate several kinetic parameters describing transport between compartments, the most important being K_i (or K_{bone}) reflecting the net clearance to bone mineral and K_1 (or K_{total}) reflecting clearance to total bone tissue and approximating blood flow.[4]

The mechanisms of ^{18}F-fluoride accumulation in the skeleton differ greatly from other tumor-specific PET radiopharmaceuticals that have been used to detect skeletal metastases. These radiopharmaceuticals include ^{18}F-fluorodeoxyglucose (^{18}FDG)[15] and ^{18}F-choline (^{18}FC),[16,17] which are tumor-specific agents with uptake reflecting metabolism in the tumor cells of a metastasis rather than reflecting the bone response as with ^{18}F-fluoride.

CLINICAL STUDIES

Early clinical assessments of ^{18}F-fluoride for detecting skeletal metastases in the 1990s were performed on PET scanners, but subsequent studies used PET/CT with the advantage of being able to combine both functional and morphologic information. Further studies have compared ^{18}F-fluoride PET as a bone-specific technique with tumor-specific tracers, including ^{18}FDG and ^{18}FC.

The early clinical studies using ^{18}F-fluoride PET were performed by Schirrmeister and colleagues.[18] An initial study prospectively assessed ^{18}F-fluoride PET in 44 patients with prostate, thyroid, or lung cancer and compared it with ^{99m}Tc–methylene diphosphonate (MDP) planar bone scintigraphy. A panel of reference methods were used as the gold standard, including radiographs, CT, MRI, and iodine 131 scintigraphy. ^{18}F-fluoride PET proved more accurate in detecting skeletal metastases than bone scintigraphy (area under receiver operating characteristic (ROC) curves 0.99 and 0.64, respectively). These results were on a lesion-by-lesion basis, but on a patient-by-patient basis the differences were less dramatic. Forty-four patients were correctly defined as positive for skeletal metastases by ^{18}F-fluoride PET compared with 42 by planar bone scintigraphy. The improved accuracy for individual lesions seemed to depend on anatomic site, with the greatest advantage for ^{18}F-fluoride seen in the spine and pelvis. The sensitivity of ^{18}F-fluoride PET was the same for osteoblastic prostate cancer metastases as it was for osteolytic metastases from lung and thyroid carcinomas. ^{18}F-fluoride PET also led to an increase in specificity compared with planar bone scintigraphy, with the ability to correctly categorize more benign and malignant lesions. This increase was thought to be due to the better anatomic localization possible with PET compared with planar scintigraphy.

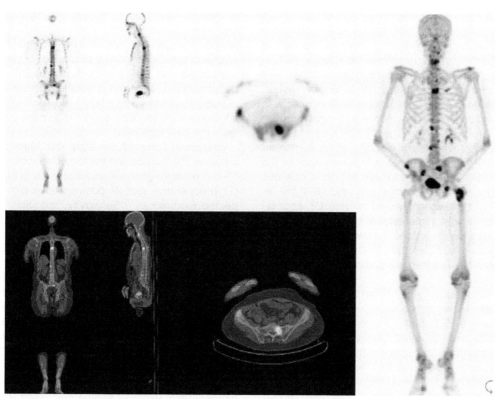

Fig. 2. A 18F-fluoride PET/CT scan of a patient with metastatic prostate cancer. Coronal, sagittal, and axial PET data (*top row*). Fused PET/CT data (*bottom row*). MIP PET image (*far right*).

A similar subsequent study from the same group evaluated 18F-fluoride PET in patients with breast cancer.[19] 18F-fluoride PET showed a better diagnostic accuracy than planar bone scintigraphy on a lesion-by-lesion basis (area under ROC 0.99 and 0.74, respectively) and patient-by-patient basis (1.0 and 0.82, respectively). A change in management resulted from detection of metastases in 4 of 34 patients with 18F-fluoride PET compared with the management strategy that was used with bone scintigraphy.

The weakness of the comparisons in these studies was that only planar scintigraphy was used and so there was an inherent advantage for the PET technique that produces tomographic images routinely. This was addressed in a subsequent study of 53 patients with lung cancer in which 18F-fluoride PET was compared with planar bone scintigraphy augmented with single-photon emission computed tomography (SPECT) of the spine.[20] Of the 12 patients with bone metastases, 6 had false-negative results with planar scintigraphy, 1 with planar scintigraphy augmented with spinal SPECT, and none with 18F-fluoride PET. There was not a significant difference in the area under the ROC curve between SPECT and PET (0.944 and 0.993, respectively). Clinical

management was changed in 5 and 6 patients as a result of the SPECT and PET findings, respectively. These findings suggested that the differences between 99mTc-MDP and 18F-fluoride imaging were largely technical rather than biologic. A subsequent larger study of 103 patients with lung cancer compared 18F-fluoride PET with planar bone scintigraphy and planar scintigraphy augmented with SPECT of the spine.[21] In this larger study, of the 33 patients with bone metastases, 13 had false-negative results with planar bone scintigraphy, 4 with SPECT, and 2 with PET. A statistical difference was found in the area under the ROC curves (0.771, 0.875, and 0.989, respectively). A change in management resulted in 8 patients due to SPECT and in 10 due to PET. A cost-effectiveness analysis was also undertaken that showed that the additional costs for each correctly diagnosed patient were 1272 Euro for SPECT and 2861 Euro for PET.

In a more recent study, 18F-fluoride PET was compared with 18FDG PET/CT and planar bone scintigraphy in 126 patients with non–small cell lung cancer.[22] In this group of patients, more skeletal metastatic lesions were detected with 18FDG PET/CT than with 18F-fluoride PET overall (53 vs 40), but there were 4 patients in whom metastases were detected only with ^{18}F-fluoride. In view of this finding, although [18]FDG PET/CT was more accurate than bone scintigraphy, it remains uncertain whether it can also replace ^{18}F-fluoride PET in staging the skeleton in lung cancer.

In one of the first studies evaluating hybrid ^{18}F-fluoride PET/CT in patients with cancer with a variety of primary tumors, the additional morphologic information from the CT component significantly improved the specificity when compared with ^{18}F-fluoride PET alone.[23] Ninety-four of the 111 metastases corresponded to lytic or sclerotic changes on the CT component, and 16 of the remaining 17 lesions showed normal CT appearances. In only 1 metastasis did PET/CT falsely suggest a benign lesion. The low-dose CT component was of sufficient quality that a full diagnostic CT was not required for correlative purposes in most lesions.

A subsequent study from the same group compared planar bone scintigraphy, SPECT, ^{18}F-fluoride PET, and ^{18}F-fluoride PET/CT in 44 patients with prostate cancer.[24] SPECT was more sensitive and specific than planar scintigraphy, and ^{18}F-fluoride PET was more sensitive than SPECT. ^{18}F-fluoride PET/CT was also more sensitive and specific than planar and SPECT bone scintigraphy. As in the previous study, the additional morphologic information from the CT component led to an increase in specificity when compared with ^{18}F-fluoride PET alone, and there were fewer equivocal interpretations. Three of the 25 patients with a new diagnosis of prostate cancer had bone metastases detected with ^{18}F-fluoride PET/CT that were not detected with planar scintigraphy, leading to a change in management to systemic rather than local therapy.

In view of the different mechanisms of uptake of ^{18}F-fluoride and [18]FDG in skeletal metastases, some researchers have postulated combining the 2 tracers to optimize diagnostic accuracy.[25,26] In the earlier study, [18]FDG and ^{18}F-fluoride were injected simultaneously (300 MBq and 100 MBq, respectively) and compared with control group who only had [18]FDG administered. Correlation with other imaging findings occurred in 88% of the combined group and 78% of the control group. This was not a statistically significant difference, but interobserver agreement in lesion localization improved from 0.74 in the control group to 0.95 in the combined group. To some extent, the better skeletal or soft tissue localization that resulted from this study has been superseded by combined PET/CT.

The later study compared [18]FDG, ^{18}F-fluoride, and combined [18]FDG/^{18}F-fluoride PET/CT scans in patients with varied cancers. Development of an image-processing algorithm in a mouse model allowed images of only the combined tracer uptake in the skeleton to be produced. These corresponded well with the ^{18}F-fluoride PET scans performed as a separate acquisition. This method allowed separate interpretation of the [18]FDG and ^{18}F-fluoride distribution even though the tracers were injected together.

Interesting comparisons have also been made between ^{18}F-fluoride and the tumor-specific agent [18]FC in prostate cancer in an initial study of 38 men (17 preoperative and 21 postoperative with suspected recurrence).[16] Sensitivity, specificity, and accuracy for ^{18}F-fluoride were 81%, 93%, and 86%, respectively and for [18]FC, 74%, 99%, and 85%, respectively. The differences in specificity were statistically significant in keeping with the tumor-specific nature of [18]FC uptake compared with nonspecific bone uptake of ^{18}F-fluoride. [18]FC PET led to a change in management in 2 patients with bone metastases not detected by ^{18}F-fluoride. This change was assumed to be due to early bone marrow detection. Although more metastases were detected with ^{18}F-fluoride in other patients, this did not change management. Sclerotic lesions with higher density as measured by CT Hounsfield units (HU) tended to be negative with both tracers, and there was a negative correlation between standard uptake values (SUV) and HU measurements. A subsequent study explored the relationship of [18]FC with CT density further.[17] An HU level greater than 825 was associated with the absence of uptake, and most of these patients were receiving hormone therapy. This suggests that the lesions may have been rendered inactive by the treatment and that a healing sclerotic response was responsible for the high density on CT. A longitudinal study would obviously be of interest in exploring this relationship further.

At the time of writing, a multicentre study is underway in the United States to assess the use of ^{18}F-fluoride PET in routine use of skeletal staging in cancer.[27] This study proposes to compare ^{18}F-fluoride PET/CT with ^{99m}Tc-MDP bone scintigraphy in 500 patients with breast, prostate, and non–small cell lung cancers. This large collaborative project will be of great interest in answering any remaining questions regarding skeletal staging with ^{18}F-fluoride.

Moving on from just using ^{18}F-fluoride for skeletal staging, there are some early data suggesting that ^{18}F-fluoride can be used to assess treatment response in prostate cancer. A small pilot study of patients with metastatic prostate cancer confined to skeleton being treated with [223]Ra-chloride used ^{18}F-fluoride PET at 6 and 12 weeks.[28] Although serial scans showed no subjective difference in uptake, it was possible to differentiate responders from nonresponders, as determined by prostate-specific antigen response, by measurement of serial SUVs. It remains to be seen whether this quantitative approach works as well in other cancers and with different types of therapy.

SUMMARY

^{18}F-fluoride PET is a highly sensitive method for the detection of skeletal metastases, and the diagnostic accuracy is further improved with ^{18}F-fluoride PET/CT where the morphologic CT information allows a further increase in specificity. As a bone-specific tracer, the use of ^{18}F-fluoride has been successfully described in a variety of cancers that produce predominantly lytic or sclerotic metastases. There are early data comparing ^{18}F-fluoride with other PET tumor-specific agents, including ^{18}FDG and ^{18}FC, showing a complementary role. It is possible that the clinical use of ^{18}F-fluoride PET/CT will continue to grow, especially if the shortage of ^{99m}Tc increases.

REFERENCES

1. Galasko CSB. The anatomy and pathways of skeletal metastases. In: Weiss L, Gilbert AH, editors. Bone metastases. Boston: GK Hall; 1981. p. 49–63.
2. Rubens RD. Bone metastases—incidence and complications. In: Rubens RD, Mundy GR, editors. Cancer and the skeleton. London: Martin Dunitz; 2000. p. 33–42.
3. Blau M, Nagler W, Bender MA. Fluorine-18: a new isotope for bone scanning. J Nucl Med 1962;3: 332–4.
4. Blake GM, Park-Holohan SJ, Cook GJR, et al. Quantitative studies of bone with the the use of ^{18}F-fluoride and ^{99m}Tc-methylene diphosphonate. Semin Nucl Med 2001;31:28–49.
5. Toegel S, Hoffman O, Wadsak W, et al. Uptake of bone seekers is solely associated with mineralisation. A study with ^{99m}Tc MDP, ^{153}Sm EDTMP and ^{18}F-fluoride on osteoblasts. Eur J Nucl Med Mol Imaging 2006;33:491–4.
6. Messa C, Goodman WG, Hoh CK, et al. Bone metabolic activity measured with positron emission tomography and [18F]fluoride ion in renal osteodystrophy: correlation with bone histomorphometry. J Clin Endocrinol Metab 1993;77:949–55.
7. Wootton R, Dore C. The single-passage extraction of 18F in rabbit bone. Clin Phys Physiol Meas 1986;7: 333–43.
8. Bang S, Baud CA. Topographical distribution of fluoride in iliac bone of a fluoride-treated osteoporotic patient. J Bone Miner Res 1990;5(Suppl 1):S87–9.
9. Narita N, Kato K, Nakagaki H, et al. Distribution of fluoride concentration in the rat's bone. Calcif Tissue Int 1990;46:200–4.
10. Grant FD, Fahey FH, Packard AB, et al. Skeletal PET with 18F-fluoride: applying new technology to an old tracer. J Nucl Med 2008;49:68–78.
11. Petren-Mallmin M, Andreasson I, Liunggren O, et al. Skeletal metastases from breast cancer: uptake of 18F-fluoride measured with PET in correlation with CT. Skeletal Radiol 1998;27:72–6.
12. Administration of Radioactive Substances Advisory Committee. Notes for guidance on the clinical administration of radiopharmaceuticals and use of sealed radioactive sources. Chilton (UK): Health Protection Agency; 2006.
13. Brenner W, Vernon C, Muzi M, et al. Comparison of different quantitative approaches to ^{18}F-fluoride PET scans. J Nucl Med 2004;45:1493–500.
14. Hawkins RA, Huang YC, Hoh CK, et al. Evaluation of the skeletal kinetics of Fluorine-18-fluoride ion with PET. J Nucl Med 1992;33:633–42.
15. Hsu WK, Virk MS, Feeley BT, et al. Characterisation of osteolytic, osteoblastic and mixed lesions in a prostate cancer mouse model using ^{18}FDG and ^{18}F-fluoride PET/CT. J Nucl Med 2008;49:414–21.
16. Beheshti M, Vali R, Waldenberger P, et al. Detection of bone metastases in patients with prostate cancer by ^{18}F fluorocholine and ^{18}F fluoride PET/CT: a comparative study. Eur J Nucl Med Mol Imaging 2008;35:1766–74.
17. Beneshti M, Vali R, Waldenberger P, et al. The use of F-18 choline PET in the assessment of bone metastases in prostate cancer: correlation with morphological changes on CT. Mol Imaging Biol 2009;11: 446–54.
18. Schirrmeister H, Guhlmann A, Elsner K, et al. Sensitivity in detecting osseous lesions depends on anatomic localization: planar bone scintigraphy versus ^{18}F PET. J Nucl Med 1999;40:1623–9.
19. Schirrmeister H, Guhlmann A, Kotzerke J, et al. Early detection and accurate description of extent of metastatic bone disease in breast cancer with fluoride ion and PET. J Clin Oncol 1999;17:2381–9.
20. Schirrmeister H, Glatting G, Hetzel J, et al. Evaluation of the clinical value of planar bone scans, SPECT and ^{18}F-labeled NaF PET in newly diagnosed lung cancer. J Nucl Med 2001;42:1800–4.
21. Hetzel M, Arslandemir C, Konig HH, et al. F-18 NaF PET for detection of bone metastases in lung cancer: accuracy, cost-effectiveness and impact on patient management. J Bone Miner Res 2003;18:2206–14.
22. Kruger S, Buck AK, Mottaghy FM, et al. Detection of bone metastases in patients with lung cancer: 99mTc MDP planar bone scintigraphy, 18F-fluoride

PET or 18F-FDG PET-CT. Eur J Nucl Med Mol Imaging 2009;36:1807–12.

23. Even-Sapir E, Metser U, Flusser G, et al. Assessment of malignant skeletal disease: initial experience with ^{18}F-fluoride PET/CT and comparison between ^{18}F-fluoride PET and ^{18}F-fluoride PET/CT. J Nucl Med 2004;45:272–8.

24. Even-Sapir E, Metser U, Mishani E, et al. The detection of bone metastases in patients with high risk prostate cancer: [99m]Tc MDP planar bone scintigraphy, single and multi field of view SPECT, ^{18}F-fluoride PET and ^{18}F-fluoride PET/CT. J Nucl Med 2006;47:287–97.

25. Hoegerle S, Juengling F, Otte A, et al. Combined FDG and F-18 fluoride whole body PET: a feasible two in one approach to cancer imaging. Radiology 1998;209:253–8.

26. Iaguru A, Mittra E, Yaghoubi SS, et al. Novel strategy for a cocktail ^{18}F-fluoride and ^{18}F-FDG PET/CT scan for evaluation of malignancy: results of the pilot phase study. J Nucl Med 2009;50:501–5.

27. Available at: http://www.ami-imaging.org/index.php?option=com_content@task=view@id=173&;Itemid=119. Accessed February 25, 2010.

28. Cook G, Parker C, Chua S, et al. Quantitative 18F-fluoride PET to monitor response in skeletal metastases from prostate cancer treated with Alpharadin (223-Ra-chloride). Nucl Med Commun 2009;30:374.

FDG PET for the Detection of Bone Metastases: Sensitivity, Specificity and Comparison with Other Imaging Modalities

Colleen M. Costelloe, MD[a],*, Hubert H. Chuang, MD, PhD[b], John E. Madewell, MD[a]

KEYWORDS

• FDG • PET • Bone • Metastases

The development of bone metastases has a major effect on the prognosis and treatment of cancer patients with solid malignancies. [^{18}F]Fluorodeoxyglucose (FDG) PET has revolutionized the imaging of many cancers and plays an increasingly important role in the detection of osseous metastases. Many imaging modalities such as radiography, computed tomography (CT), skeletal scintigraphy (SS; bone scan), single-photon emission tomography (SPECT), and magnetic resonance (MR) imaging are also used for the detection of bony metastases and have various strengths and weaknesses compared with FDG PET imaging. A PubMed search of the English literature was performed using the keywords "PET," "metastasis," and "bone" from January 1, 2000 to January 1, 2010. Separate searches in the same time frame included the terms "PET, metastasis" and "x-ray," "skeletal survey," "whole body MRI," and "bone scan." "PET, bone, SPECT" and "PET, CT, metastasis" were also searched. The studies in **Tables 1–5** provided sensitivity and specificity data exclusive to detection of bone metastases, and all values were required to be greater than 0. This article reviews the sensitivity and specificity of FDG PET compared with other imaging modalities for the detection of osseous metastases in solid malignancies.

Radiography is an x-ray–based technology that images the calcified structure of bone. Calcium is found in the cortex and, to a lesser extent, in the trabecular bone of the medullary cavity. Osseous metastases can be classified as lytic, sclerotic, or mixed at initial presentation and lytic metastases tend to heal with rim and internal sclerosis.[1] Radiography is relatively insensitive for the detection of osseous metastases. Most lesions arise in the medullary cavity and many must enlarge to the extent that they destroy more than 50% of the cortex before they can be detected on radiographs.[2,3] This results in a delay in detection while the tumor enlarges to the degree that it produces sufficient cortical destruction. It can take 4 to 12 months for osseous metastases to become visible on radiography.[4]

Blastic metastases increase bone density. Although blastic metastases are generally easier to detect than lytic metastases in the axial skeleton, the overlap of anatomic structures is often a confounding factor for the detection of both

[a] Division of Diagnostic Imaging, Department of Diagnostic Radiology, The University of Texas MD Anderson Cancer Center, 1515 Holcombe Boulevard, Houston, TX 77030, USA
[b] Division of Diagnostic Imaging, Department of Nuclear Medicine, The University of Texas MD Anderson Cancer Center, 1515 Holcombe Boulevard, Houston, TX 77030, USA
* Corresponding author.

PET Clin 5 (2010) 281–295
doi:10.1016/j.cpet.2010.04.001

Table 1
PET compared with CT

Author	Tumor	Patients	Reference Standard	Bone Metastases	Sensitivity PET (%)	Specificity PET (%)	Sensitivity CT (%)	Specificity CT (%)
Liu et al[38,a]	Cervix	356	Biopsy or FU 180 d	29 patients	93.3	99.5	33.3	99.1
Mahner et al[7,b]	Breast	119	Biopsy or mean FU 11 mo	32 patients	87	92	67	95
Median (%)	—	—	—	—	90.1	95.8	50.2	97.1

Unless stated otherwise, the follow-up (FU) period for all studies included imaging, possible clinical information, and was conducted for a minimum of the recorded length of time.
[a] The study by Liu et al[38] also compared PET with conventional MRI, as is mentioned in the text.
[b] The study by Maher et al[7] also provided data on the sensitivity and specificity of radiography and SS (see **Table 2**).

Table 2
PET compared with SS

Author	Tumor	Patients	Bone Metastases	Reference Standard	Sensitivity PET (%)	Specificity PET (%)	Sensitivity SS (%)	Specificity SS (%)
Kato et al[19]	Esophagus	44	31 in 13 patients	Biopsy or FU 6 mo	92	94	77	84
Gayed et al[24]	Lung	85	82 patients	FU mean 7.9 mo	73	88	81	78
Ito et al[47]	Thyroid	47	67 in 18 patients	Imaging at time of study	84.7	99.6	78.0	91.4
Liu et al[48]	Endemic Nasopharyngeal	202	30 patients	FU 1 y	70.0	98.8	36.7	97.7
Kim et al[49]	Head and neck	564	17[a]	Biopsy, FU 6 mo	87.8	99.6	78.0	99.7
Abe et al[23]	Breast	44	14 patients[a]	Biopsy, FU 6 mo	84.4	98.6	80.0	98.6
Ohta et al[20]	Breast	51	9 patients	Biopsy, FU 1 y	77.7	97.6	77.7	80.9
Gallowitsch et al[50]	Breast	62	135	Biopsy, FU mean 24 mo	56.5	88.9	89.8	74.1
Mahner et al[7,b]	Breast	119	32 patients	Biopsy, mean FU 11 mo	87	92	67	99
Dose et al[51]	Breast	50	12	FU mean 12.6 mo	83.3	89.4	88.8	91.6
Median (%)	—	—	—	—	83.9	95.8	78.0	91.5

Unless stated otherwise, the follow-up (FU) period for all studies included imaging, possible clinical information, and was conducted for a minimum of the recorded length of time.
Abbreviation: SS, skeletal scintigraphy.
[a] Presented data are based on anatomic regions.
[b] The study by Mahner et al also provided data on the sensitivity and specificity of radiography (discussed in text) and CT (see Table 1).

Table 3
PET/CT compared with SS

Author	Tumor	Patients	Bone Metastases	Reference Standard	Sensitivity PET (%)	Specificity PET (%)	Sensitivity SS (%)	Specificity SS (%)
Min et al[30]	Lung	182	30 patients	Biopsy, average FU 333 d	93.3	94.1	93.3	44.1
Takenaka et al[42,a]	Lung	137	67 25 patients	Biopsy, FU 12 mo	97.0	95.4	95.5	95.0
Median (%)	—	—	—	—	95.2	94.6	94.2	69.8

Unless stated otherwise, the follow-up (FU) period for all studies included imaging, possible clinical information, and was conducted for a minimum of the recorded length of time.

Abbreviation: SS, skeletal scintigraphy.

[a] This study also provided data for whole-body (WB) MRI (Table 5).

Table 4
PET and PET/CT compared with conventional imaging (CI; SS and some combination of radiography, diagnostic CT, or MRI)

Author	Tumor	Patients	Bone Metastases	Reference Standard	Sensitivity PET (%)	Specificity PET (%)	Sensitivity CI (%)	Specificity CI (%)
Yoon et al[34,a]	Hepatocellular	87	11	FU 3 mo	100	100	45.5	100
Ng et al[35,b]	Nasopharyngeal	111	9	Biopsy, FU 12 mo	88.9	98.0	22.2	99.0
Median (%)	—	—	—	—	94.5	99.0	33.9	99.5

Unless stated otherwise, the follow-up (FU) period for all studies included imaging, possible clinical information, and was conducted for a minimum of the recorded length of time.
[a] PET alone.
[b] PET/CT.

Table 5
PET/CT compared with WB MRI

Author	Tumor	Patients	Bone Metastases	Reference Standard	Sensitivity PET (%)	Specificity PET (%)	Sensitivity MRI (%)	Specificity MRI (%)
Takenaka et al[42,a]	Lung	137	67 25 patients	Biopsy, FU 12 mo	97.0	95.4	73.1	96.4
Schmidt et al[43,b]	Various	30	102 23 patients	FU 6 mo	78.0	80.0	94.0	76.0
Antoch et al[52]	Various	98	75, 80[c]	Biopsy, FU mean 273 d	62	96	85	92
Median (%)	—	—	—	—	78.0	95.4	85.0	92.0

Unless stated otherwise, the follow-up (FU) period for all studies included imaging, possible clinical information, and was conducted for a minimum of the recorded length of time.
[a] This study also provided the data for SS in Table 3.
[b] No intravenous contrast was administered on the WB MRI.
[c] The total number of patients with bone metastases and the total number of bone metastases were not given. There were 75 true-positive lesions found in 8 patients on PET/CT and 80 true-positive lesions found in 11 patients on WB MRI.

types of lesion. Despite its limitations, radiography is extremely specific for the diagnosis of osseous metastases. This makes radiography useful when coupled with imaging modalities that are more sensitive than specific, such as SS.[5,6]

Throughout this article the term PET is used for PET alone without fused CT. Fused studies are referred to as PET/CT, and FDG PET is referred to as PET for the remainder of the article. No dedicated studies comparing PET or PET/CT with radiography were discovered in the literature search. A study by Mahner and colleagues[7] compared radiography, CT, SS, and PET for the detection of osseous metastases and provided separate sensitivity and specificity data for each modality. The study included 32 breast cancer patients with bone metastases and the sensitivity and specificity of PET were 87% and 92%, compared with 57% and 100% for radiography. PET was found to be more sensitive than radiography, but had a lower specificity, and the investigators did not comment on whether this difference was significant. The specificity of radiography was 100%. If a lesion is seen on radiographs, it can usually be diagnosed as metastatic disease with a high degree of confidence. Aside from issues of cost and availability, the high sensitivity of PET makes this modality suitable as an initial screening tool. PET imaging can be augmented by radiography or CT, particularly if an integrated PET/CT scanner is used.

CT is an x-ray–based technology that provides detailed calcium imaging and is extremely sensitive for the detection of blastic metastases. The nature of tomographic imaging aids lesion detection by eliminating overlap from other structures in the axial skeleton. A lesser degree of cortical lysis is necessary for the detection of lytic metastases on CT compared with radiography, but the soft-tissue contrast resolution of CT is limited. Therefore, noncalcified tumor that has not grown large enough to significantly affect the cortex is often not clearly visible in the medullary cavity unless it destroys a large degree of trabecular bone or is surrounded by dark, fatty marrow. Although soft-tissue windowing can be helpful, bone windowing is generally superior for the detection of lytic or sclerotic metastases. Bone windowing can also help characterize other findings, such as fractures and benign bone tumors (eg, enchondromas and fibrous dysplasia),[8] and it is recommended that the skeleton be viewed with bone and soft-tissue windows.

The studies in **Table 1** compare the sensitivity and specificity of PET with diagnostic CT for the detection of bone metastases. The results indicate that PET is more sensitive than CT (median 90.1% and 50.2%, respectively) with similar specificity (median 95.8% and 97.1%, respectively). Separate from and in addition to the data presented in **Table 1**, the study conducted by Mahner and colleagues[7] also performed a direct comparison between PET and CT (implying that the information in **Table 1** and other data sets was based on the strong study design of isolated evaluation of each imaging modality rather than side-by-side comparisons). The sensitivity and specificity of CT did not change (67% and 95% respectively), whereas the sensitivity and specificity of PET became 92% and 86% respectively. Although not statistically different from the data in **Table 1**, the specificity of CT in the direct comparison was found to be higher than PET. The high sensitivity of PET and high specificity of CT is a basis for fused PET/CT imaging.

A prospective multicenter study comparing PET with diagnostic CT in melanoma patients with palpable nodal metastases conducted by Bastiaannet and colleagues[9] brings up a practical issue regarding the interpretation of CT while evaluating for bone metastases. More bony metastases were detected on PET than CT ($P<.0001$) but many of the lesions were found on CT in retrospect, suggesting that the readers of the diagnostic CT scans did not use bone windowing. Bone window settings provide increased image contrast and are essential for the detection of many subtle lesions.

Klies and colleagues[10] investigated PET/CT, PET, and CT in 43 patients with pediatric solid malignancies. A detailed investigation of the size of detected lesions was performed regarding all 3 imaging modalities. PET/CT detected 5 lesions of less than 5 mm and 66 lesions larger than 5 mm. PET detected 0 lesions less than 5 mm and 30 lesions larger than 5 mm whereas CT detected 5 lesions less than 5 mm and 58 lesions larger than 5 mm. Fused PET/CT was more efficacious in detecting lesions of both sizes, particularly compared with PET alone. Additionally, the investigators pointed out a pitfall in the detection of marrow metastases. Red, hematopoietic marrow is diffusely FDG avid and normally found throughout the skeleton of children. Red marrow activity can obscure metastases on PET and MRI. rendering metastatic foci only visible on radiography, CT (lysis or sclerosis), or bone scan. In the adult population this does not typically occur because red marrow regresses to the axial skeleton and diminishes in cellularity with advancing age.[11] Red marrow hypertrophy can nevertheless occur throughout the adult skeleton following the administration of cytokines (eg, colony stimulating factors), which are used to correct cytopenia associated with chemotherapy or other causes.[12] Therefore, different patterns of marrow uptake can be seen. Heterogeneous FDG avidity is often caused by metastases[13] that can be obscured by red marrow hypertrophy at a different time point, as described earlier. The cause of diffuse homogeneous marrow uptake can be benign or malignant (lymphoma, leukemia) and can be investigated through a review of the medical history or by bone marrow biopsy.

SS is used to detect bony metastases through the mechanism of diphosphonate tracers, such as technetium (Tc) 99m methylene diphosphonate (MDP) and Tc 99 m hydroxymethylene diphosphonate (HMDP), that bind to the hydroxyapetite produced by the bone as it attempts to repair damage caused by metastatic tumor.[14] In rapidly growing or purely lytic metastases, this healing response may not occur to an extent that it is detectable by SS. Malignancies that typically produce this type of metastasis (renal cell, thyroid carcinoma, and multiple myeloma) are often a source of false-negative results on bone scan. Otherwise, SS is typically sensitive, but not as specific, for the detection of osseous metastases.[5,15] Many conditions other than metastatic

disease can result in tracer uptake, such as degenerative or arthritic joint disease and trauma. Therefore, bone scan is often coupled with radiography to produce a sensitive and specific method of imaging bony metastases.[1,16,17]

The studies in **Table 2** compare the sensitivity and specificity of PET with SS for the detection of bony metastases. A larger number of studies were found comparing PET with bone scan (n = 10, see **Table 2**) than with CT (n = 2, see **Table 1**), and a greater degree of variability was reported for the sensitivity of PET in **Table 2** (56.5%–92%) than in **Table 1** (87.0% – 93.3%). This result more likely reflects variations in the studies, such as size or methodology (eg, per-lesion, per-region or per-patient comparisons), than in the sensitivity of PET for the detection of osseous metastases. The median sensitivity of PET in **Table 2** was higher than that of bone scan (83.9% and 78%, respectively, **Fig. 1**). The specificity of PET (88%–99.6%, median 95.8%) was similar to or higher than that of SS (74.1%–99.7%, median 91.5%). PET is a powerful tool for imaging the skeleton and it has been suggested by the American Society of Clinical Oncology that bone scan is optional for the staging of lung cancer in patients with evidence

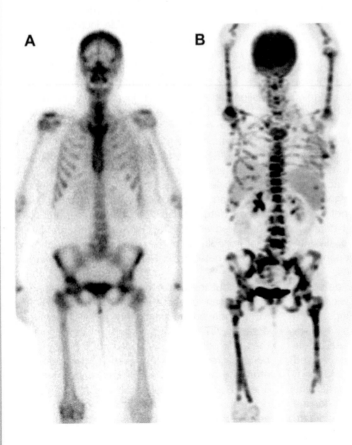

A   B

Fig. 1. Superior sensitivity of PET compared with SS in a patient with breast cancer. (*A*) Tc 99m MDP bone scan was interpreted as abnormal regarding a subtle prominence of activity in the humeri and femora consistent with bone metastases (the lower legs were normal and have been cropped to allow better visualization of the remainder of the examination). No metastases were seen in the axial skeleton. (*B*) Maximum intensity projection FDG PET image obtained the same day shows widespread bony metastases in the appendicular and axial skeleton. In this example, PET was more sensitive for the detection of osseous metastases than SS.

of bone metastases on PET, with the exception of painful areas that are not included in the PET field of view.[18]

In addition to evaluating the efficacy of PET for detecting bony metastases, the studies conducted by Kato and colleagues[19] (see **Table 2**) and Ohta and colleagues[20] (see **Table 2**) suggest that PET can detect metastatic lesions earlier than SS. An example of this concept is found in the study performed by Kut and colleagues[21] of small-cell lung cancer patients. The investigators studied 21 patients, some of whom had PET studies before therapy plus during/after therapy with comparison with CT or bone scan. PET detected a metastasis to the spine 4 weeks before SS or CT, and PET also revealed an additional spinal lesion that was not evident on the comparison bone scan but was detected on subsequent bone scans. Most imaging modalities detect the change in bone caused by the tumor rather than the tumor itself. By reflecting the metabolism of the tumor cells, it is reasonable that some lesions should be detectable earlier with PET than with other techniques.

FDG activity was compared with morphologic findings on CT in a study conducted by Du and colleagues[22] that included 146 bone metastases in 25 patients with breast cancer who received serial PET/CT scans. Eighteen patients had prior systemic therapy and 14 had radiation therapy,

but not closer than 4 weeks before the initial PET/CT scans. At baseline, 93.5% (n = 72) of the lytic, 81.8% (n = 9) of the mixed, and 61% (n = 25) of the blastic lesions were FDG avid. The difference in maximum standardized uptake value (SUV_{max}) between lytic and blastic lesions was not significant ($P = .2$). Seventeen lesions without CT findings were diagnosed as bone metastases on the basis of FDG uptake. Seven patients had received no prior therapy. In these patients, 27/28 lytic and 16/17 blastic lesions were FDG avid on baseline PET/CT.

Following therapy, 80.5% (n = 58) of the lytic lesions became sclerotic and non–FDG avid (**Fig. 2**). Loss of FDG avidity occurred more rapidly than sclerosis, which was often gradual, sometimes occurring over a period of more than 2 years. The investigators report that the sclerosis was unaffected by the type of anticancer therapy used (many patients received hormonal, chemotherapy, or radiation therapy following the baseline scans). Approximately half of the mixed lesions remained FDG avid. All of the 17 PET-positive and CT-negative lesions became non–FDG avid, and 9 of them developed sclerosis on the CT. Thirteen of the 25 blastic lesions became non–FDG avid following therapy. The other 12 remained avid and increased in size on CT, presumably indicating disease progression. A limited comparison was also made with bone scan. One-hundred and eight

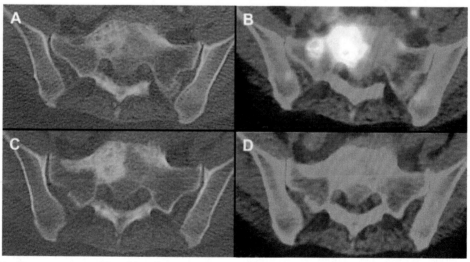

Fig. 2. Healing response on CT and fused PET/CT images in a patient with breast cancer. (*A*) CT portion of a PET/CT examination in bone windows shows a mixed lytic/sclerotic lesion on the right side of the S1 segment. (*B*) Companion fused PET/CT image shows FDG activity consistent with an active metastatic lesion. (*C*) Sclerosis has occurred in the lesion on the CT portion of a PET/CT performed 7 months later. (*D*) Companion fused image shows resolution of FDG uptake. Effectively treated lytic and mixed bony metastases often heal with sclerosis and loose FDG avidity. If the second examination was the patient's baseline, this lesion could be mistaken for a nonavid blastic metastasis rather than a treated lesion. Review of the patient's treatment history is important when interpreting the appearance of bone metastases.

of the 146 metastases identified on PET/CT were detected on bone scan and most of them continued to be positive on follow-up bone scans. The investigators conclude that this study indicates that FDG uptake reflects the immediate tumor activity of bone metastases. PET could potentially reveal positive therapeutic response more quickly than CT or bone scan.

The patients in the study conducted by Abe and colleagues[23] (see **Table 2**) received hormonal therapy but no chemotherapy before the investigation. Nine lesions were false-negative on SS, and the investigators note that they tended to occur in patients with diffuse marrow metastases or lytic lesions. A further comparison was made between lytic and blastic metastases. PET detected 14/19 blastic metastases, whereas bone scan detected 17/19. Of the lytic metastases, PET detected 24/26, whereas bone scan detected 19/26. PET is likely more efficacious than bone scan for the detection of lytic lesions because of a relative paucity of reparative bone formation in some of the metastases.

The study by Gayed and colleagues[24] brought up an issue of spatial resolution on PET studies. The investigators found that bone scan was able to differentiate between the presence or absence of rib invasion in 3 patients with lung cancer, whereas PET was indeterminate for the presence of adjacent bony lesions. The ambiguity of PET in this situation is understandable because the FDG uptake of the tumor would be contiguous with rib activity, but MDP could separate the structures by localizing preferentially to bone rather than tumor. This is an example of a situation in which PET/CT imaging would likely resolve the indeterminate findings rendered by PET alone. The investigators comment that the sensitivity (73%) and positive predictive value (46%) of PET (see **Table 2**) were lower than other published values and suggest that this may be explained by inaccurate localization of bone lesions to soft tissues, which is another phenomenon that could largely be corrected with fused PET/CT imaging.

The studies in **Table 3** compare the sensitivity and specificity of PET/CT with bone scan for the detection of osseous metastases. The median sensitivity of fused PET/CT is higher in **Table 3** (95.2%) compared with the results of the studies of PET alone (83.9%, see **Table 2**), whereas median specificity is high for both (94.6% and 95.8%, respectively). Compared with bone scan, PET/CT has similar sensitivity and higher specificity (median 95.2% and 94.6% for PET/CT and 94.2% and 69.8% for bone scan, respectively).

Nagaoka and colleagues[25] compared PET/CT with PET alone and bone scan in a prospective study of 21 patients with hepatocellular or combined hepatocellular/cholagniocarcinoma. Bone metastases were discovered in 4 patients with a total of 16 lesions. Bone scan revealed 11 of the lesions. Five of the metastases not detected on bone scan were seen on PET, and fused PET/CT revealed all of the lesions. Therefore, PET/CT was most sensitive, followed by PET alone, and bone scan was the least sensitive for the detection of bone metastases in this patient population. Although the sensitivity of PET is low for the detection of primary hepatocellular carcinoma[26] (particularly regarding well-differentiated tumors),[27] it could potentially be helpful for detecting distant metastases.[28,29]

The study by Min and colleagues[30] showed a higher specificity with PET/CT (94.1%) than SS (44.1%) (see **Table 3**), which the investigators attributed to the high anatomic resolution of the fused CT. Nevertheless, this study mentions a problematic issue regarding the increased sensitivity of PET/CT. Two patients with bone lesions were found in the spine on the CT portion of the examination that were not found on bone scan and were not FDG avid. The investigators state that the efficacy of PET/CT could not be demonstrated in this situation, presumably due to ambiguity regarding the benign or malignant nature of the lesions. Numerous potential confounding factors can occur in the spine. For example, endplate defects, also known as Schmorl nodes, can be caused by benign herniation of disc material into the vertebral body or by the focal collapse of bone compromised by metastatic deposits. MRI is the optimal imaging modality for assessing the extent of tumor in the marrow cavity[31] and may be helpful in situations in which CT findings are ambiguous and must be further investigated.

Ak and colleagues[32] conducted a retrospective study of 95 non–small-cell lung cancer patients and discovered 19 patients with FDG-avid bone metastases but negative bone scans (20% of the population). The PET/CT examinations revealed lytic lesions. This study exemplifies the previously discussed phenomenon of increased sensitivity of PET for lytic lesions that do not produce sufficient reparative bone response to be detected on SS.

SPECT can be used to perform SS in an axial fashion, thereby improving lesion detection and identification through increased contrast resolution. The mechanism of action of diphosphonate tracers is the same as in planar bone scan, and SPECT is susceptible to many of the same pitfalls. One applicable study was found during the literature search. Uematsu and colleagues[33] evaluated 15 breast cancer patients with 900 bone metastases. The sensitivity and specificity of PET for detection of the lesions was 17% and 100%, whereas the values for SPECT were 85% and 99%. The reference standard was sound, requiring detection of each abnormality on at least 1 other imaging modality with a follow-up period of more than 12 months. Seven patients were evaluated for initial staging and 8 for restaging with 3 patients previously known to have bone metastases. The treatment status of the patients was not specifically mentioned. The reported PET sensitivity value of 17% is the lowest in this review and it can be postulated that treatment status may have played a role. Regarding morphology, PET detected 9/143 blastic and 18/20 lytic metastases. Bone SPECT detected 132/143 blastic and 7/20 lytic metastases. Following the trend previously seen on comparison of planar bone scan with PET, the PET scans were found to be superior to SPECT regarding the detection of lytic metastases. Conversely, SPECT was more sensitive than PET for the detection of sclerotic metastases. FDG PET and SS (planar or SPECT) seem to be complementary regarding the detection of lytic versus blastic bone metastases.

The studies by Yoon and colleagues[34] and Ng and colleagues[35] in **Table 4** compared PET and PET/CT respectively with a combination of conventional imaging (CI) studies such as radiography, diagnostic CT, or MRI. When comparing the PET results with each other, the sensitivity of PET and PET/CT is high (100% and 88.9%, respectively). That the sensitivity of PET/CT seems lower than PET alone may be secondary to differences in tumor histology or small sample size. The specificity of both was similar and high (100% and 98%, respectively). Compared with CI, the PET modalities were found to be more sensitive (median 94.5% compared with 33.9% for CI) and equally specific (median 99.0% and 99.5% for CI). The high sensitivity of PET is generally complementary to other imaging modalities for the detection of bone metastases.

MRI produces diagnostic images by manipulating the spin of free protons in tissue. When placed in a strong magnetic field, the spins have a useful tendency to line up with the field. Energy is added in the form of radiofrequency pulses, flipping the protons into desired orientations. After a brief interval, the spins return to their original states and energy is given off in the form of radio frequency waves that are intercepted by the magnet's receiver coil, producing an electric current from which images are generated. MRI has the capability of producing the greatest soft-tissue contrast resolution of any modern imaging technique and provides exquisite soft-tissue detail of the medullary cavity of bone. Because bone

metastases typically originate in the medullary cavity, MRI can detect them early.[36,37] For the purposes of this review, conventional MRI is defined as MRI performed over a limited coverage area using pulse sequences typical for regional rather than whole-body (WB) imaging. WB MRI is mentioned later.

One study in this review compared PET with conventional MRI. Liu and colleagues[38] evaluated 29 patients with cervical cancer and bone metastases. Comparison was made between PET, CT (see **Table 1**), and conventional MRI. The sensitivity and specificity of PET were 94.1% and 99.1%, respectively. The values for conventional MRI were 70.6% and 96.1%, respectively. The results of a receiver operating curve indicated that the diagnostic performance of PET was superior to those of CT ($P<.001$) and MRI ($P = .033$) (**Fig. 3**).

WB (WB) MR coverage is becoming feasible through the use of specialized WB MRI techniques. Traditional MRI is limited to specific anatomic regions because of the lengthy nature of traditional pulse sequences and the increase in artifacts that occurs when scanning large areas of anatomy. Through the use of fast pulse sequences that are resistant to these artifacts, multiplanar, multisequence, WB acquisitions can be achieved in approximately 1 hour.[39] WB MRI has been shown to be superior to SS for the detection of bony metastases[40,41] and may replace SS for routine WB skeletal survey in the future.[17] All of the WB MRI studies included in this review include intravenous gadolinium contrast unless otherwise specified.

The studies in **Table 5** compare the sensitivity and specificity of PET/CT with WB MRI for the detection of bony metastases. The sensitivity and specificity of PET/CT (median 78.0% and 95.4%) and WB MRI (median 85.0% and 92.0%) are generally high with a trend toward higher sensitivity with WB MRI. The high sensitivity of MRI is expected considering its excellent marrow soft-tissue resolution. Whole-body cancer staging with PET/CT and WB MRI is an active field of investigation at the time of this review, and more studies evaluating the role of these modalities in the detection of osseous metastases are expected in the near future.

Separate from and in addition to the data in **Table 5** (which are for WB MRI performed with typical WB pulse sequences), the study by Takenaka and colleagues[42] also evaluated WB diffusion-weighted (DW) MRI. Combined with more typical WB MRI pulse sequences (eg, T1 gradient echo, short tau inversion recovery [STIR]), sensitivity increased to 95.5% (from 73.1%) and specificity

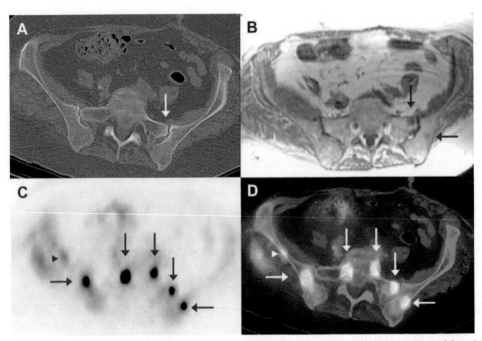

Fig. 3. Comparison of CT, MRI, PET, and PET/CT in a patient with angiosarcoma. (*A*) CT portion of fused PET/CT study shows mild sclerosis on the sacral side of the left sacroiliac joint that could represent degenerative change (*arrow*). (*B*) MRI performed the day before the PET/CT shows metastases in the left iliac wing and the left poster-omedial iliac bone (*arrows*). (*C*) PET alone reveals 5 foci of FDG uptake suspicious for metastases (*arrows*) with a questionable sixth lesion in the right lateral pelvis (*arrowhead*). Incidental note is made of FDG uptake in the right gluteal musculature that is associated with a displaced right hip arthroplasty (not shown). (*D*) The fused PET/CT of (*A*) and (*C*) provides specificity by localizing the suspicious foci to bone rather than lymph nodes or other structures (*arrows*). The equivocal focus of uptake in the right lateral pelvis (*arrowhead*) localizes to the right iliac bone and is likely another osseous metastasis. Functional imaging was more sensitive for the detection of bone metastases than anatomic imaging in this example, and the CT provided specificity through anatomic localization of the suspicious foci of FDG uptake seen on the PET-only image.

stayed the same (96.1% from 96.4%). DW imaging has been shown to be useful in the brain for detecting acute ischemia and is being investigated for oncologic indications in numerous organ systems. More investigation is needed to determine the usefulness of this promising technique in the detection of bony metastases.

The study by Schmidt and colleagues[43] conducted in 2007 (see **Table 5**) apparently used the typical PET/CT coverage area of skull base to upper thighs. WB MRI coverage extended from the top of the skull to the feet. Because of the limited PET coverage area, 10 more lesions were discovered on WB MRI than on PET/CT (1 mandible, 7 distal femora, 2 tibias). The investigators do not mention whether any of these metastases were solitary and would, therefore, change patient staging. Nevertheless, the presence of metastases can predispose to pathologic fracture if the lesions are lytic, with serious clinical implications for mastication or weight bearing. Problematic metastases can be treated with limited surgical procedures or radiation therapy if found

before fracture, whereas larger surgical procedures are often necessary after fracture occurs, which is a powerful argument for extending the coverage of PET/CT in cancer patients. These investigators also found that WB MRI was more sensitive than PET/CT for the detection of lesions less than 1 cm in size (88% compared with 56%, respectively). This finding was attributed to the high tissue contrast resolution of MRI, particularly on STIR sequences.

A study of various malignancies by Schmidt and colleagues,[44] conducted in 2005, also compared the efficacy of WB MRI and PET for the detection of osseous metastases. WB MRI detected 76 bone metastases compared with 50 with PET/CT. Similarly, WB MRI also detected more bony metastases than PET/CT in a different study conducted by this group comparing 1.5 T, 3 T WB MRI with PET/CT in 2008.[45] The investigators of the 2005 study compared the size of the lesions on each imaging modality and found that the size of the bone metastases detected on MRI ranged from 2 to 50 mm, with a median size of 17 mm.

The size of bone metastases detected on PET/CT ranged from 9 to 50 mm with a median of 27 mm. These results suggest that WB MRI is better able to detect smaller lesions than PET/CT.

Most of the WB MRI studies in this review compare PET/CT with whole-body MRI, reflecting the recent development of WB MRI. A study conducted by Ohno and colleagues[46] investigated PET alone compared with WB MRI. Ninety lung cancer patients with 25 bone metastases were included. The reference standard was biopsy or imaging follow-up for approximately 2 years. PET was found to have a sensitivity of 88.0% and specificity of 88.3%. The values for WB MRI were 88.0% and 96.1%, respectively. WB MRI had higher specificity (96.1%) and accuracy (94.8%) than PET (88.3% and 88.2%). Specificity was more equivalent between PET/CT and WB MRI in **Table 5** (median 95.4% and 92.0%, respectively), likely reflecting the influence of fused CT on the detection of bone metastases

SUMMARY

As a functional, WB imaging modality, FDG PET plays an important role in the detection of bony metastases. Many studies have found PET to have higher sensitivity for the detection of osseous metastases compared with other imaging modalities. A potential exception is when comparing PET with bone scan in the setting of blastic metastases. Most lytic bone lesions heal with sclerosis, and FDG activity is expected to decrease or resolve following effective treatment. These factors may contribute to the apparent deficiency of PET in this regard. It has been postulated that the cellularity of sclerotic lesions is less than that of lytic lesions and may be less than the threshold for detection by PET. Several studies have found the same lesions to be simultaneously negative on PET but positive on SS, suggesting that bone remodeling may continue for an extended period. Therefore, PET may be a better indicator of active bony metastases.

Compared with the large number of studies comparing PET alone with other imaging modalities for the detection of bone metastases, there is a paucity of studies that perform the same comparisons with fused PET/CT and provide sensitivity and specificity data. Increased specificity is expected as a result of the excellent anatomic localization provided by fused PET/CT imaging, allowing the exclusion of nonmalignant sources of FDG uptake. More studies using fused PET/CT for the detection of osseous metastases are needed to clarify the potential advantages of fused imaging in this regard.

PET/CT retains certain limitations, such as the poor soft-tissue contrast resolution of CT that limits evaluation of the marrow cavity. Modalities such as MRI have been found capable of detecting smaller bone metastases than PET/CT. Ongoing research comparing PET/CT with WB MRI is expected to further clarify the strengths, weaknesses, and clinical usefulness of these WB studies for the detection of osseous metastases.

PET imaging has been shown to be useful for the detection of bone metastases. PET alone tends to be more sensitive than most other imaging modalities, and the efficacy of PET can be increased with companion or fused anatomic imaging.

REFERENCES

1. Hamaoka T, Madewell JE, Podoloff DA, et al. Bone imaging in metastatic breast cancer. J Clin Oncol 2004;22:2942–53.
2. Galasko CS. Skeletal metastases and mammary cancer. Ann R Coll Surg Engl 1972;50:3–28.
3. Edelstyn GA, Gillespie PJ, Grebbell FS. The radiological demonstration of osseous metastases. Experimental observations. Clin Radiol 1967;18:158–62.
4. Cook GJ, Fogelman I. Skeletal metastases from breast cancer: imaging with nuclear medicine. Semin Nucl Med 1999;29:69–79.
5. Hortobagyi GN, Libshitz HI, Seabold JE. Osseous metastases of breast cancer. Clinical, biochemical, radiographic, and scintigraphic evaluation of response to therapy. Cancer 1984;53:577–82.
6. Perez DJ, Powles TJ, Milan J, et al. Detection of breast carcinoma metastases in bone: relative merits of X-rays and skeletal scintigraphy. Lancet 1983;2:613–6.
7. Mahner S, Schirrmacher S, Brenner W, et al. Comparison between positron emission tomography using 2-[fluorine-18]fluoro-2-deoxy-D-glucose, conventional imaging and computed tomography for staging of breast cancer. Ann Oncol 2008;19:1249–54.
8. Costelloe CM, Murphy WA Jr, Chasen BA. Musculoskeletal pitfalls in 18F-FDG PET/CT: pictorial review. AJR Am J Roentgenol 2009;193:WS1–13 [quiz S26–30].
9. Bastiaannet E, Wobbes T, Hoekstra OS, et al. Prospective comparison of [18F]fluorodeoxyglucose positron emission tomography and computed tomography in patients with melanoma with palpable lymph node metastases: diagnostic accuracy and impact on treatment. J Clin Oncol 2009;27:4774–80.
10. Kleis M, Daldrup-Link H, Matthay K, et al. Diagnostic value of PET/CT for the staging and restaging of

pediatric tumors. Eur J Nucl Med Mol Imaging 2009; 36:23–36.

11. Ellis RE. The distribution of active bone marrow in the adult. Phys Med Biol 1961;5:255–8.

12. Kazama T, Swanston N, Podoloff DA, et al. Effect of colony-stimulating factor and conventional- or high-dose chemotherapy on FDG uptake in bone marrow. Eur J Nucl Med Mol Imaging 2005;32:1406–11.

13. Chiang SB, Rebenstock A, Guan L, et al. Diffuse bone marrow involvement of Hodgkin lymphoma mimics hematopoietic cytokine-mediated FDG uptake on FDG PET imaging. Clin Nucl Med 2003;28:674–6.

14. Arano Y. Recent advances in 99 mTc radiopharmaceuticals. Ann Nucl Med 2002;16:79–93.

15. Loeffler RK, DiSimone RN, Howland WJ. Limitations of bone scanning in clinical oncology. JAMA 1975; 234:1228–32.

16. Corcoran RJ, Thrall JH, Kyle RW, et al. Solitary abnormalities in bone scans of patients with extra-osseous malignancies. Radiology 1976;121:663–7.

17. Costelloe CM, Rohren EM, Madewell JE, et al. Imaging bone metastases in breast cancer: techniques and recommendations for diagnosis. Lancet Oncol 2009;10:606–14.

18. Pfister DG, Johnson DH, Azzoli CG, et al. American Society of Clinical Oncology treatment of unresectable non-small-cell lung cancer guideline: update 2003. J Clin Oncol 2004;22:330–53.

19. Kato H, Miyazaki T, Nakajima M, et al. Comparison between whole-body positron emission tomography and bone scintigraphy in evaluating bony metastases of esophageal carcinomas. Anticancer Res 2005;25:4439–44.

20. Ohta M, Tokuda Y, Suzuki Y, et al. Whole body PET for the evaluation of bony metastases in patients with breast cancer: comparison with 99Tcm-MDP bone scintigraphy. Nucl Med Commun 2001;22:875–9.

21. Kut V, Spies W, Spies S, et al. Staging and monitoring of small cell lung cancer using [18F]fluoro-2-deoxy-D-glucose-positron emission tomography (FDG-PET). Am J Clin Oncol 2007;30:45–50.

22. Du Y, Cullum I, Illidge TM, et al. Fusion of metabolic function and morphology: sequential [18F]fluoro deoxyglucose positron-emission tomography/computed tomography studies yield new insights into the natural history of bone metastases in breast cancer. J Clin Oncol 2007;25:3440–7.

23. Abe K, Sasaki M, Kuwabara Y, et al. Comparison of 18FDG-PET with 99 mTc-HMDP scintigraphy for the detection of bone metastases in patients with breast cancer. Ann Nucl Med 2005;19:573–9.

24. Gayed I, Vu T, Johnson M, et al. Comparison of bone and 2-deoxy-2-[18F]fluoro-D-glucose positron emission tomography in the evaluation of bony metastases in lung cancer. Mol Imaging Biol 2003;5:26–31.

25. Nagaoka S, Itano S, Ishibashi M, et al. Value of fusing PET plus CT images in hepatocellular carcinoma and combined hepatocellular and cholangiocarcinoma patients with extrahepatic metastases: preliminary findings. Liver Int 2006;26:781–8.

26. Delbeke D, Martin WH, Sandler MP, et al. Evaluation of benign vs malignant hepatic lesions with positron emission tomography. Arch Surg 1998;133:510–5 [discussion: 515–6].

27. Trojan J, Schroeder O, Raedle J, et al. Fluorine-18 FDG positron emission tomography for imaging of hepatocellular carcinoma. Am J Gastroenterol 1999;94:3314–9.

28. Khan MA, Combs CS, Brunt EM, et al. Positron emission tomography scanning in the evaluation of hepatocellular carcinoma. J Hepatol 2000;32:792–7.

29. Torizuka T, Tamaki N, Inokuma T, et al. In vivo assessment of glucose metabolism in hepatocellular carcinoma with FDG-PET. J Nucl Med 1995;36:1811–7.

30. Min JW, Um SW, Yim JJ, et al. The role of whole-body FDG PET/CT, Tc 99 m MDP bone scintigraphy, and serum alkaline phosphatase in detecting bone metastasis in patients with newly diagnosed lung cancer. J Korean Med Sci 2009;24:275–80.

31. Zimmer WD, Berquist TH, McLeod RA, et al. Bone tumors: magnetic resonance imaging versus computed tomography. Radiology 1985;155:709–18.

32. Ak I, Sivrikoz MC, Entok E, et al. Discordant findings in patients with non-small-cell lung cancer: absolutely normal bone scans versus disseminated bone metastases on positron-emission tomography/computed tomography. Eur J Cardiothorac Surg 2010;37(4):792–6.

33. Uematsu T, Yuen S, Yukisawa S, et al. Comparison of FDG PET and SPECT for detection of bone metastases in breast cancer. AJR Am J Roentgenol 2005;184:1266–73.

34. Yoon KT, Kim JK, Kim do Y, et al. Role of 18F-fluorodeoxyglucose positron emission tomography in detecting extrahepatic metastasis in pretreatment staging of hepatocellular carcinoma. Oncology 2007;72(Suppl 1):104–10.

35. Ng SH, Chan SC, Yen TC, et al. Staging of untreated nasopharyngeal carcinoma with PET/CT: comparison with conventional imaging work-up. Eur J Nucl Med Mol Imaging 2009;36:12–22.

36. Colman LK, Porter BA, Redmond J 3rd, et al. Early diagnosis of spinal metastases by CT and MR studies. J Comput Assist Tomogr 1988;12:423–6.

37. Algra PR, Bloem JL, Tissing H, et al. Detection of vertebral metastases: comparison between MR imaging and bone scintigraphy. Radiographics 1991;11:219–32.

38. Liu FY, Yen TC, Chen MY, et al. Detection of hematogenous bone metastasis in cervical cancer: 18F-fluorodeoxyglucose-positron emission tomography versus computed tomography and magnetic resonance imaging. Cancer 2009;115:5470–80.

39. Ma J, Costelloe CM, Madewell JE, et al. Fast Dixon-based multisequence and multiplanar MRI for whole-body detection of cancer metastases. J Magn Reson Imaging 2009;29:1154–62.

40. Engelhard K, Hollenbach HP, Wohlfart K, et al. Comparison of whole-body MRI with automatic moving table technique and bone scintigraphy for screening for bone metastases in patients with breast cancer. Eur Radiol 2004;14:99–105.

41. Eustace S, Tello R, DeCarvalho V, et al. A comparison of whole-body turboSTIR MR imaging and planar 99 mTc-methylene diphosphonate scintigraphy in the examination of patients with suspected skeletal metastases. AJR Am J Roentgenol 1997; 169:1655–61.

42. Takenaka D, Ohno Y, Matsumoto K, et al. Detection of bone metastases in non-small cell lung cancer patients: comparison of whole-body diffusion-weighted imaging (DWI), whole-body MR imaging without and with DWI, whole-body FDG-PET/CT, and bone scintigraphy. J Magn Reson Imaging 2009;30:298–308.

43. Schmidt GP, Schoenberg SO, Schmid R, et al. Screening for bone metastases: whole-body MRI using a 32-channel system versus dual-modality PET-CT. Eur Radiol 2007;17:939–49.

44. Schmidt GP, Baur-Melnyk A, Herzog P, et al. High-resolution whole-body magnetic resonance image tumor staging with the use of parallel imaging versus dual-modality positron emission tomography-computed tomography: experience on a 32-channel system. Invest Radiol 2005;40: 743–53.

45. Schmidt GP, Baur-Melnyk A, Haug A, et al. Comprehensive imaging of tumor recurrence in breast cancer patients using whole-body MRI at 1.5 and 3 T compared to FDG-PET-CT. Eur J Radiol 2008; 65:47–58.

46. Ohno Y, Koyama H, Nogami M, et al. Whole-body MR imaging vs. FDG-PET: comparison of accuracy of M-stage diagnosis for lung cancer patients. J Magn Reson Imaging 2007;26:498–509.

47. Ito S, Kato K, Ikeda M, et al. Comparison of 18F-FDG PET and bone scintigraphy in detection of bone metastases of thyroid cancer. J Nucl Med 2007;48: 889–95.

48. Liu FY, Chang JT, Wang HM, et al. [18F]fluoro-deoxyglucose positron emission tomography is more sensitive than skeletal scintigraphy for detecting bone metastasis in endemic nasopharyngeal carcinoma at initial staging. J Clin Oncol 2006;24:599–604.

49. Kim MR, Roh JL, Kim JS, et al. 18F-fluorodeoxyglucose-positron emission tomography and bone scintigraphy for detecting bone metastases in patients with malignancies of the upper aerodigestive tract. Oral Oncol 2008;44:148–52.

50. Gallowitsch HJ, Kresnik E, Gasser J, et al. F-18 fluorodeoxyglucose positron-emission tomography in the diagnosis of tumor recurrence and metastases in the follow-up of patients with breast carcinoma: a comparison to conventional imaging. Invest Radiol 2003;38:250–6.

51. Dose J, Bleckmann C, Bachmann S, et al. Comparison of fluorodeoxyglucose positron emission tomography and "conventional diagnostic procedures" for the detection of distant metastases in breast cancer patients. Nucl Med Commun 2002;23:857–64.

52. Antoch G, Vogt FM, Freudenberg LS, et al. Whole-body dual-modality PET/CT and whole-body MRI for tumor staging in oncology. JAMA 2003;290: 3199–206.

Whole-body MRI for Detecting Bone Marrow Metastases

Thomas C. Kwee, MD[a],*, Taro Takahara, MD, PhD[a],
Kazuhiro Katahira, MD, PhD[b], Katsuyuki Nakanishi, MD, PhD[c]

KEYWORDS
- Whole-body • Magnetic resonance imaging • MRI
- Bone marrow • Metastases

Cancer is a major public health problem in the United States and many other parts of the world. This is reflected in the high number of new cancer cases (1,479,350) and the 562,340 deaths from cancer that are projected to occur in the United States in 2009.[1] The bone marrow is a common site for metastasis in cancer.[1] For example, autopsy studies have shown that bone marrow metastases can be found in approximately 70% of patients with prostate or breast cancer and in approximately 35% to 40% of patients with renal, lung, or thyroid cancer.[2] Accurate detection of (the number of) bone marrow metastases is of crucial importance because of its therapeutic and prognostic implications.[2] Furthermore, timely recognition and subsequent treatment of bone marrow metastases may prevent or reduce associated complications, such as pain, hypercalcemia, pathologic fractures, compression of the spinal cord or cauda equina, and spinal instability.[2]

Cancer cells are lodged in the bone marrow as the initial site for skeletal metastasis by means of hematogenous spread. In addition, bone marrow metastases are most frequently localized in the hematopoietic (red) marrow because of its richer blood supply compared with fatty (yellow) marrow. Consequently, the localization of bone marrow metastases is dependent on the distribution of the red marrow. At birth, visually, all marrow is of the red type. Conversion of red to yellow marrow

begins in the postnatal period, first in the extremities, progressing from the peripheral toward the axial skeleton and from diaphysis to the metaphysis of individual long bones. By the age of 25 years, marrow conversion is usually complete, and red marrow is predominantly seen in the axial skeleton and in the proximal part of the appendicular skeleton. Consequently, in adults, the most common sites for bone marrow metastases are the vertebrae (69%), pelvis (41%), proximal femoral metaphyses (25%), and skull (14%).[3,4] A study in 62 patients (mean age: 64 years; age range: 33–87 years) with metastatic bone disease, however, showed that although 60% of bone lesions were located in the axial skeleton, 40% were located in the appendicular skeleton (**Fig. 1**).[5] In this series of patients, most lesions in the appendicular skeleton were asymptomatic.[5] In children, the expected rate of bone marrow metastases in the appendicular skeleton is even higher because they have higher amounts of red marrow in this part of the skeleton. For these reasons, there is a need for a diagnostic test that allows (1) direct visualization of metastatic lesions in the bone marrow and (2) assessment of the bone marrow throughout the entire body.

Commonly used diagnostic tests for the detection of bone (marrow) metastases include bone marrow biopsy (BMB) and imaging modalities, such as conventional radiography, CT, and bone

[a] Department of Radiology, University Medical Center Utrecht, Heidelberglaan 100, Utrecht 3584 CX, The Netherlands
[b] Department of Radiology, Kumamoto Central Hospital, 1-5-1, Tainoshima, Kumamoto-shi, Kumamoto 862-0965, Japan
[c] Department of Radiology, Osaka Medical Center for Cancer and Cardiovascular Diseases, 1-3-3 Nakamichi, Higashinari-ku, Osaka 537-8511, Japan
* Corresponding author.
E-mail address: thomaskwee@gmail.com

PET Clin 5 (2010) 297–309
doi:10.1016/j.cpet.2010.03.006
1556-8598/10/$ – see front matter © 2010 Elsevier Inc. All rights reserved.

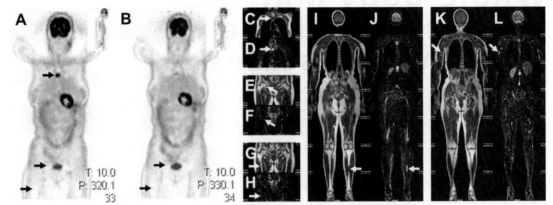

Fig. 1. ^{18}F-FDG–PET and whole-body MRI in a 71-year-old woman with Waldenström macroglobulinemia and bone metastatic disease. Coronal ^{18}F-FDG–PET images (A, B) show foci with increased ^{18}F-FDG uptake in the sternal manubrium, right acetabulum, and right femur (arrows), indicating bone marrow metastases. The same lesions are seen on coronal T1-weighted (C, E, G) and STIR (D, F, H) images of the whole-body MRI examination; the low signal intensity (comparable to muscle) on T1-weighted images and the high signal intensity on STIR images is highly suggestive for bone marrow metastases. Coronal T1-weighted (I, K) and STIR (J, L) whole-body MRI-detected additional bone marrow metastases in the left tibia (I, J) (arrows) and in the right humerus (J, L) (arrows). FDG-PET could not depict these lesions because they were outside its field of view.

scintigraphy. BMB has a high specificity, but it is an invasive and painful procedure with a small but non-negligible risk of (hemorrhagic) complications.[6] Furthermore, a BMB allows evaluation of only a limited portion of the entire bone marrow. Consequently, BMB is prone to sampling errors and has a limited sensitivity.[7] Conventional radiography is inexpensive and widely available. Although conventional radiography is of great value in the assessment of cortical and trabecular bone,[8] it yields projection images only, and a change of 30% to 50% in mineral density is needed before a bone lesion becomes visible.[9] Consequently, sensitivity for the detection of small lesions may be impaired.[10,11] CT provides cross-sectional images, allows for whole-body imaging, is suitable to visualize cortical and trabecular bone, and is more sensitive than conventional radiography.[10,11] A significant limitation of CT, however, is that it is not suitable for bone marrow assessment. Furthermore, the considerable radiation that is associated with CT is a non-negligible issue.[12] Bone scintigraphy is frequently performed to screen for bone metastatic disease in patients with a proved malignancy. Metastases confined to the bone marrow and metastases that do not induce any osteoblastic reaction, however, are missed by bone scintigraphy. Moreover, conventional planar and single-photon emission CT images have limited spatial resolution, which further impairs sensitivity.[13,14]

Two other cross-sectional imaging modalities that may be of value for the assessment of bone marrow metastases are MRI[15,16] and PET.[13,14,17]

MRI allows direct visualization of all bone marrow components at a good spatial resolution.[15,16] Furthermore, technologic advances, including the development of high-performance magnetic field gradients, parallel imaging, faster MRI sequences, and new coil and table concepts, have made MRI of the entire body clinically feasible. PET can be performed using a wide variety of radiotracers, including ^{18}F-fluoride and ^{18}F-fluoro-2-deoxyglucose (^{18}F-FDG).[18] The use of ^{18}F-FDG–PET may be of particular value, because it directly images tumor cells based on their metabolic activity.[13,14,17] When using a state-of-the-art combined PET/CT system, whole-body PET imaging can be performed in 20 minutes or less. Furthermore, the CT component of a PET/CT study facilitates anatomic localization of sites with abnormal radiotracer uptake, thereby improving diagnostic performance. An important advantage of whole-body MRI and FDG-PET compared with conventional radiography, CT, and bone scintigraphy is their ability to visualize bone marrow metastases at an early stage, before bone remodelling has occurred.[13–17] This article reviews whole-body MRI techniques and the diagnostic performance of whole-body MRI compared with PET for the detection of bone marrow metastases.

WHOLE-BODY MRI TECHNIQUES
Anatomic Coverage and Imaging Planes

In routine clinical practice, MRI is usually performed as a second-line imaging modality after conventional radiography or bone scintigraphy.

Furthermore, MRI is a useful method to evaluate skeletal causes of neurologic symptoms in patients with known cancer. In these situations, the MRI examination is limited to the body region of interest, and bone marrow metastases outside the image volume are missed. Whole-body MRI allows assessment of metastases throughout the entire bone marrow but is different from MRI examinations of limited body regions in that it allows less time to acquire different MRI sequences and imaging planes and generally uses a greater slice thickness and lower spatial resolution. Although there is no widely agreed-on method for detecting bone marrow metastases using whole-body MRI, whole-body MRI is usually performed or displayed in the coronal plane. The field of view should provide complete anterior-to-posterior coverage per station, and the number of stations should at least cover the skull, vertebrae, pelvis, and proximal femoral metaphyses.[3,4] Nevertheless, complete superior-to-inferior body coverage (ie, from vertex to heels) is preferable (see **Fig. 1**), especially in children.[3,4] It is also recommended to acquire sagittal images of the spine to improve evaluation of the vertebrae, discs, and spinal cord.

Whole-body MRI Sequences

There is no consensus yet which (combination of) whole-body MRI sequences provides the highest diagnostic yield while being time efficient. Nevertheless, commonly used whole-body MRI sequences that can be considered as indispensable for the evaluation of the bone marrow are T1-weighted and fat-saturated T2-weighted or short inversion time inversion recovery (STIR) sequences.[19,20] On T1-weighted images, yellow marrow (composed of 80% fat, 15% water, and 5% proteins[16]) exhibits a high signal intensity that is approximately similar to that of subcutaneous fat. Red marrow (composed of 40% fat, 40% water, and 20% proteins[16]) is hypointense compared with yellow marrow, although its signal intensity is still greater than that of muscle. On fat-saturated T2-weighted and STIR images, signal of yellow marrow is almost nulled, whereas signal of red marrow is hyperintense. Bone marrow metastases typically have longer T1 and T2 relaxation times than normal yellow and red marrow (ie, low signal intensity on T1-weighted images and high signal intensity of fat-saturated T2-weighted or STIR images), because they contain larger amounts of water and lesser amounts of fat. In general, MRI can be regarded as a sensitive technique for the detection of bone marrow metastases. Its specificity, however, may be suboptimal.[21] In particular, the discrimination between reconverted or red marrow (islands) and bone marrow metastases may sometimes be difficult due to overlap in signal intensities.[15,16] Furthermore, osteoblastic metastases may have shorter T2 relaxation times, as a result of which their signal intensity may be diminished on fat-saturated T2-weighted and STIR images. Specific MRI signs have been proposed to improve the diagnosis of bone marrow metastases.[22] One MRI sign is called the bull's-eye sign. This sign is different from the bull's eye sign on ultrasonography, which is suggestive of liver metastasis. In contrast, this bull's eye sign was reported a specific indicator of normal red marrow (sensitivity, 95%; specificity, 99.5%). It refers to the presence of 1 or more foci of high signal intensity (equivalent to subcutaneous fat) within an area of low signal intensity on T1-weighted imaging, reflecting (converted) fatty marrow within a region of (reconverted) red marrow. In addition to the bull's eye-sign, bilateral symmetric or diffuse hypersignal intensities on fat-suppressed T2-weighted and STIR images are also highly suggestive of normal red marrow. Another MRI sign is a positive sign for osteoblastic metastasis. It is called the halo sign and refers to the presence of a rim with high signal intensity around a lesion with lower signal intensity on T2-weighted imaging. The outer layer corresponds to peritumoral edema and the central core corresponds to the tumor itself. The halo sign and the presence of diffuse signal hyperintensity on T2-weighted imaging have been reported to be strong indicators of bone metastatic disease (sensitivity, 75%; specificity, 99.5%).[22]

Gadolinium-enhanced T1-weighted images can improve the detection of bone marrow metastases; normal marrow usually shows no visible contrast enhancement, whereas bone marrow metastases often exhibit strong signal increase. If gadolinium-enhanced T1-weighted images are acquired, it is important to compare them with noncontrast-enhanced T1-weighted images (by means of side-by-side viewing or by creating subtracted images), because enhancing lesions may mimic yellow marrow, which is originally hyperintense. Another way to overcome this problem is by acquiring gadolinium-enhanced T1-weighted images with fat saturation, which suppresses yellow marrow. On the other hand, the addition of gadolinium-enhanced sequences prolongs scan time of a whole-body MRI examination. Furthermore, STIR imaging has been reported to be at least equal to gadolinium-enhanced MRI for the detection of bone marrow lesions.[23,24] For these reasons, it can be argued that gadolinium-enhanced sequences may be omitted from a whole-body MRI examination for the detection of bone marrow metastases.

In addition to conventional MRI sequences, diffusion-weighted MRI (DWI) is emerging as a powerful technique for the detection of bone marrow metastases.[25–27] DWI is a fat-suppressed T2-weighted sequence that is sensitive to the random (brownian) extra-, intra-, and transcellular motion of water molecules, driven by their internal thermal energy. Yellow marrow is suppressed at DWI thanks to the use of a fat-suppression pre-pulse, whereas red marrow demonstrates higher signal intensity because of its high cellularity and water content. Because many malignant tumors, including bone marrow metastases, have a prolonged T2 relaxation time and an impeded diffusion, they often exhibit high signal intensity at DWI (equal to or higher than that of the spinal cord). One of the main advantages of DWI over conventional MRI sequences is its good lesion-to-background contrast. Nevertheless, it is important to combine DWI with conventional MRI sequences to improve lesion localization, because DWI has a low spatial resolution and lacks sufficient anatomic background information. Furthermore, the addition of conventional MRI sequences (in particular T1-weighted imaging) is necessary to improve detectability of osteoblastic metastases, which, unlike osteolytic metastases, may exhibit low signal intensity at DWI.[28] A new approach for the acquisition of whole-body diffusion-weighted images is the concept of diffusion-weighted whole-body imaging with background body signal suppression (DWIBS).[25] In DWIBS, diffusion-weighted images are acquired under free breathing. This allows increasing signal-to-noise ratio (SNR) by acquiring multiple signal averages, which allows obtaining thin slices (typically 4–5 mm). Details about this concept can be read elsewhere.[29] An important advantage of DWIBS over conventional MRI sequences and regular thick-sliced diffusion-weighted images is that acquired images can be handled as a volumetric data set. Consequently, the original DWIBS data set is suitable to create multiplanar reformats and 3-D displays, such as maximum intensity projections (Figs. 2–5). This, in turn, allows evaluating curved skeletal structures (eg, the rib cage or skull) over long trajectories, which may improve detectability of bone marrow lesions in these locations.[25–27] Previous studies[30–32] reported that coronal and sagittal T1-weighted and STIR whole-body may failed to detect bone marrow metastases in the rib cage and skull. In this context, the acquisition of a DWIBS data set may be of additional value. In a study that included 30 patients with various malignancies, reported region-based sensitivity of conventional (T1-weighted and STIR) whole-body MRI combined with whole-body DWI (96%) was significantly higher (P<.05) than that of conventional whole-body MRI alone (88%).[26] Another study, including 115 patients with non–small cell lung cancer (NSCLC),[27] reported that sensitivity and accuracy of conventional (T1-weighted and STIR) whole-body MRI combined with whole-body DWI (95.5% and 96.1%, respectively) were significantly higher (P<.05) than that of conventional whole-body MRI alone (73.1% and 94.8%, respectively). Nevertheless, although DWI may be a sensitive additional sequence for the detection of bone marrow metastases, signal intensities of bone marrow metastases and normal red marrow at DWI may overlap. DWI may also be used to follow-up patients with bone metastatic disease (see Fig. 5) and to monitor therapeutic efficacy. It has been shown that water mobility in bone metastases may show early changes as a result of treatment effects, which can be visualized and quantified using DWI.[33,34] As such, it may be a good alternative to conventional MRI, because the size criteria defined by the World Health Organization and the Response Evaluation Criteria in Solid Tumors are not suitable to assess tumor response in bone.[35] More research is warranted to validate this promising application of DWI.

To improve specificity of MRI for the detection of bone marrow metastases, in particular the differentiation between residual or reconverted red marrow (islands) and bone marrow metastases, it has been proposed to perform MRI after administration of ultrasmall particles of iron oxide (USPIOs).[36–39] Intravenously administered USPIOs are taken up by macrophages in the reticuloendothelial system, predominantly within the lymph nodes but also in red and yellow marrow.[36–39] Approximately 1 hour after administration of USPIOs, T2 relaxation times of normal red and yellow marrow are considerably lower than precontrast relaxation times. Consequently, hyperplastic or normal red marrow exhibits low signal intensity on USPIO-enhanced fat-saturated T2-weighted, STIR, and diffusion-weighted images. On the other hand, bone marrow metastases do not take up USPIOs, as a result of which their relaxation times do not decrease. Consequently, bone marrow metastases maintain high signal intensity on USPIO-enhanced fat-saturated T2-weighted, STIR, and diffusion-weighted images.[36–39] In a study including 9 patients with non-Hodgkin lymphoma who underwent non–contrast-enhanced MRI and USPIO-enhanced MRI of the spine, it was shown that contrast between bone marrow metastases

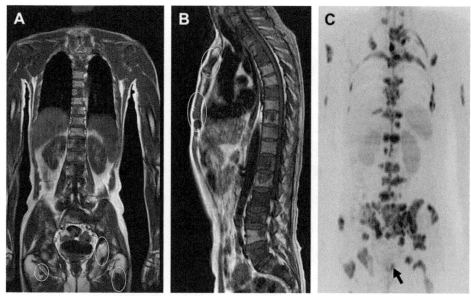

Fig. 2. Whole-body MRI, including DWI, in a 66-year-old patient with prostate cancer and bone metastases. Coronal T1-weighted image (*A*) and sagittal whole-spine T1-weighted image (*B*) show multiple foci of low signal intensity in the cervical, thoracic, lumbar, and sacral vertebral bodies, thoracic spinous processes, left ilium, bilateral femurs, and sternum (*encircled*), indicating bone marrow metastases. Coronal maximum intensity projection gray-scale inverted DWI acquired using the concept of DWIBS (*C*) shows multiple foci of high signal intensity throughout the skeleton (including humeri, rib cage, vertebral bodies, pelvic bone, and femurs) in a single view, indicating extensive bone metastatic disease. Also note that the signal intensity in the left side of the prostate gland (*arrow*) is higher than that of the contralateral side, which corresponds to the primary tumor. The normal prostate gland usually shows high signal intensity at DWI but has a low signal intensity on this image due to the applied window level/width settings.

and normal bone marrow on STIR images can be increased significantly (*P*<.05) after USPIO administration.[38] In another study in 22 patients with non-Hodgkin lymphoma (including 9 patients before and 13 patients after conditioning therapy) who underwent non–contrast-enhanced MRI and USPIO-enhanced MRI of the spine, it was reported that overall lesion detectability was significantly (*P* = .002) better on the postcontrast images compared with the precontrast images. In detail, significantly (*P* = .006) more lesions less than 1 cm were depicted on the postcontrast images, but for lesions greater than 1 cm no significance could be detected (*P* = .8).[39] Although USPIO-enhanced MRI is a promising method for the detection of bone marrow metastases, it has not yet been evaluated in larger series of patients with different primary tumors. Furthermore, the feasibility of USPIO-enhanced whole-body MRI has not been demonstrated. Another, perhaps more serious, problem is that the availability of the current generation of USPIOs is limited. Nevertheless, effectiveness and safety of a new generation of USPIOs (P904, Guerbet Laboratories, Paris, France) are being tested in preclinical studies.

Advantages of this new USPIO agent are its faster blood pharmacokinetics and the early uptake in the reticuloendothelial system. These, in turn, may decrease the necessary time between USPIO administration and actual scanning. It is expected that this new contrast agent will get approval for clinical applications within the next few years, and its application in whole-body MRI of bone marrow metastases has great potential.

Scan Procedure and Postprocessing

State-of-the-art MRI systems are equipped with a moving table platform that allows sequential scanning of separate, consecutive body levels (stations) without repositioning the patient. Furthermore, because the slice selection gradients match exactly at each station, anatomic alignment between separate stations is maintained. Postprocessing software implemented in standard clinical software packages allows the separately acquired stations to be aligned and merged into one seamless whole-body image.[40] Coil selection is an important but challenging in issue in whole-body MRI. An integrated body coil or surface coils can

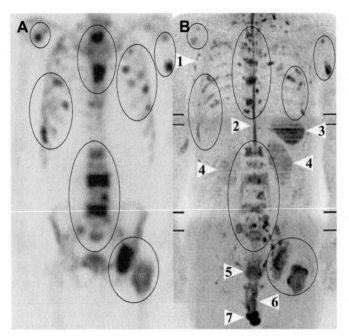

Fig. 3. Bone scintigraphy and whole-body DWI in a 75-year-old patient with prostate cancer and bone metastases. Bone scintigraphy (*A*) shows increased uptake of ^{99m}Tc-dicarboxypropane diphosphonate throughout the skeleton (including humeri, sternum, rib cage, vertebral bodies, left ilium, and left femur) (*encircled*), indicating bone metastases. Coronal maximum intensity projection gray-scale inverted DWI acquired using the concept of DWIBS (*B*) shows the same lesions as foci of high signal intensity (*encircled*), at a higher spatial resolution. Also note normal high signal intensity of axillary lymph nodes (*arrowhead 1*), spinal cord (*arrowhead 2*), spleen (*arrowhead 3*), kidneys (*arrowheads 4*), prostate gland (*arrowhead 5*), penis (*arrowhead 6*), and testes (*arrowhead 7*) at DWI.

be used for signal reception. Advantages of using an integrated body coil are that no coils have to be wrapped around the patient (which is more operator friendly and more comfortable for the patient) and the large anatomic coverage. Furthermore, it can be argued that SNR at higher magnetic field strengths, such as 3.0T, is sufficient to use an integrated body coil instead of surface coil. Alternatively, advantages of using surface coils are superior SNR or spatial resolution and the possibility of performing parallel imaging, which may be necessary for scan time reduction and which is indispensable for echo-planar imaging-based sequences, such as (whole-body) DWI. Thus, from an image quality perspective, the use of surface coils is favored. One approach that some vendors offer is the use of a so-called integrated whole-body surface coil design. A whole-body surface coil design combines a large number of seamlessly integrated coil elements and independent radiofrequency channels, which offers large anatomic coverage (approximately of 200 cm) and allows image acquisition without any time loss due to patient or coil repositioning. Setting up the different coil elements before the examination, however, is a time-consuming process that

takes several minutes. Furthermore, most MRI systems in routine clinical practice may not yet be equipped with an integrated whole-body surface coil design. Moreover, for many of these systems, an easily available upgrade toward fully integrated whole-body surface coil technology may not be available (yet). Another way to perform whole-body MRI is by using a so-called nonintegrated sliding surface coil approach.[41] The advantage of this approach is that it only requires a single surface coil with limited anatomic coverage. To perform such an examination, an additional table platform should be mounted on top of the original patient table. Furthermore, spacers should be placed between both tables to create space to move the dorsal part of the surface coil from one station to the next and so on. As a result, a patient can remain in the same position relative to the table, repositioning of the surface coil to image the next station requires only little additional time (<1 minute per station), and 3-D alignment among the imaged stations is maintained. However, such an approach is laborious. Furthermore, it narrows the bore diameter in the vertical direction by approximately 6 to 7 cm because of the use of spacers and an additional table platform, and it may not provide full

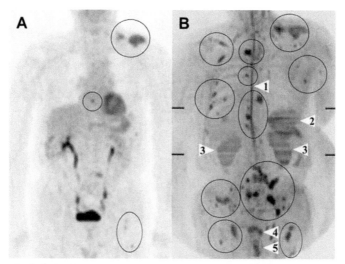

Fig. 4. ^{18}F-FDG–PET and whole-body DWI in a 73-year-old man with left-sided lung cancer (previously treated with radiotherapy) and progressive bone metastatic disease. Coronal ^{18}F-FDG–PET image (*A*) shows high ^{18}F-FDG uptake in the left clavicle, sternum, and left femur (*encircled*), indicating bone marrow metastases. Coronal maximum intensity projection gray-scale inverted DWI acquired using the concept of DWIBS, 1 month after ^{18}F-FDG–PET (*B*), shows multiple foci of high signal intensity throughout the skeleton (*encircled*), surpassing the number of lesions seen at ^{18}F-FDG–PET 1 month earlier; this may suggest progressive disease or superior sensitivity of DWI compared with ^{18}F-FDG–PET. Spatial resolution of DWI is superior to that of ^{18}F-FDG–PET. Also note normal high signal intensity of the spinal cord (*arrowhead 1*), spleen (*arrowhead 2*), kidneys (*arrowheads 3*), prostate gland (*arrowhead 4*), and penis/testes (*arrowhead 5*) at DWI.

body coverage.[41] Attempts are under way to develop a more sophisticated version of this nonintegrated sliding coil concept. Typical scan time for a whole-body MRI examination that includes coronal (non–contrast-enhanced) T1-weighted and STIR sequences of the entire body and sagittal (non–contrast-enhanced) T1-weighted and STIR sequences of the spine is currently approximately 30 minutes. If whole-body DWI (acquired using the concept of DWIBS) is also performed, total scan time can range up to 60 minutes.

WHOLE-BODY MRI COMPARED WITH PET

PubMed/MEDLINE was searched for articles comparing whole-body MRI with PET for the detection of bone marrow metastases, using the search strategy shown in **Table 1**. Studies that included patients with primary bone tumors, case reports, and studies investigating less than 10 subjects were excluded. Of 704 potentially relevant articles, 10 studies[27,32,42–49] fulfilled the selection criteria.

Heusner and colleagues[42] prospectively compared axial T1-weighted, fat-saturated T2-weighted, and fat-suppressed gadolinium-enhanced whole-body MRI at 1.5T with full-dose, contrast-enhanced ^{18}F-FDG–PET/CT for the detection of bone metastases in 54 consecutive patients with newly diagnosed NSCLC and 55 patients with newly diagnosed malignant melanoma. All tumors were ^{18}F-FDG–PET positive. Mean time interval between ^{18}F-FDG–PET/CT and whole-body MRI was 0.6 days (range, 0–11 days). Whole-body MRI and ^{18}F-FDG–PET/CT data sets were assessed by different observers who were blinded to the findings of the other imaging modality. Radiologic and clinical follow-up (mean follow-up time, 434 days; range, 42–1297 days) served as the standard of reference. Of 109 patients, 11 patients suffered from bone metastases. Patient-based sensitivity, specificity, positive predictive value (PPV), negative predictive value (NPV), and accuracy for the detection of bone metastases were 64%, 94%, 54%, 96%, and 91% for whole-body MRI, and 45%, 99%, 83%, 94%, and 94% for ^{18}F-FDG–PET/CT, without any significant differences between the 2 imaging modalities (*P* = .6147). The investigators concluded that whole-body MRI and ^{18}F-FDG–PET/CT seem equally suitable for the detection of skeletal metastases in patients suffering from newly diagnosed NSCLC and malignant melanoma. Because of a substantial rate of false-negative findings, however, modalities seem of limited value for the detection of bone metastases on initial staging of malignant melanoma and NSCLC patients with low tumor stages. Limitations of this study are the low number of patients with bone metastases, the absence of

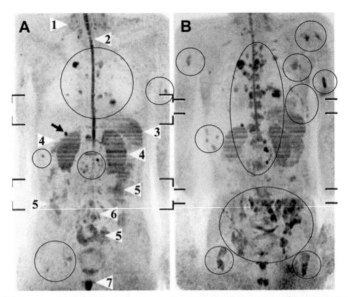

Fig. 5. Whole-body DWI as an easy and inexpensive method for the follow-up of bone metastatic disease in a 62-year-old patient with prostate cancer. Coronal maximum intensity projection gray-scale inverted DWI acquired using the concept of DWIBS (*A*) shows several foci with moderate to high signal intensity in the left humerus, rib cage, lungs, vertebra, right ilium, and femur (*encircled*), indicating widespread metastatic disease. The same type of scan 2 months later (*B*) shows a considerable increase in the number of (bone marrow) lesions (*encircled*), indicating progressive disease. Also note normal high signal intensity of the brachial plexus (*arrowhead 1*), spinal cord (*arrowhead 2*), spleen (*arrowhead 3*), kidneys (*arrowheads 4*), intestinal contents (*arrowheads 5*), lumbosacral plexus (*arrowhead 6*), and penis/testes (*arrowhead 7*) at DWI (*A*). Furthermore, (*A*) DWI also shows a (benign) sebaceous cyst (*arrow*).

histopathologic correlation, and that advanced whole-body MRI sequences, such as whole-body DWI, were not performed.[42]

Takenaka and colleagues[27] prospectively compared the diagnostic performance of coronal and sagittal in-phase (non–contrast-enhanced and gadolinium-enhanced) T1-weighted, opposed-phase T1-weighted, STIR, and diffusion-weighted whole-body MRI at 1.5T with ^{18}F-FDG–PET/CT with respect to bone metastasis assessment in 115 consecutive patients with NSCLC before treatment. All studies were performed in random order within 3 weeks of diagnosis and before treatment. Whole-body MRI and ^{18}F-FDG–PET/CT data sets were assessed by different observers who were blinded to the findings of the other imaging modality. The reference standard for the presence or absence of bone metastasis of a given site was determined based on the results of initial and follow-up bone scintigraphy, integrated ^{18}F-FDG–PET/CT, and whole-body MRI examinations and pathologic examinations from CT-guided or surgical biopsies (n = 52 sites) as well as of follow-up examinations for more than 12 months (n = 973 sites) for every patient. Of the 115 patients, 25 had bone metastases. On per-site and a per-patient bases, sensitivities of whole-body DWI alone and whole-body DWI combined

with conventional whole-body MRI were not significantly different (*P*>.05) from that of ^{18}F-FDG–PET/CT. On per-site and per-patient bases, however, specificities of whole-body DWI alone (93.7% and 78.9%, respectively) were significantly lower (*P*<.05) than those of ^{18}F-FDG–PET/CT (95.4% and 85.6%, respectively). Alternatively, specificity on a per-site basis of the combination of whole-body DWI with conventional whole-body MRI was significantly higher (*P*<.05) than that of ^{18}F-FDG–PET/CT (95.4%), with no significant differences in specificity (*P*>.05) on a per-patient basis between the 2 modalities. Takenaka and colleagues[27] concluded that whole-body MRI with DWI is more specific and accurate for the assessment of bone metastases in patients with NSCLC than ^{18}F-FDG–PET/CT. In addition, when using whole-body DWI as an adjunct to whole-body MRI without whole-body DWI, the sensitivity and accuracy of the whole-body MRI examination can be improved. This well-designed study has only some minor limitations, among which is that histopathologic results were (inevitably) not available in every patient.[27]

Laurent and colleagues[43] prospectively compared coronal gadolinium-enhanced T1-weighted, coronal STIR, and axial diffusion-weighted whole-body MRI at 1.5T with ^{18}F-FDG–PET/CT for staging advanced

Table 1 Search strategy and results from PubMed/MEDLINE as of 2 January 2010		
Step	**Search String**	**No. of Articles**
1	Magnetic resonance OR MR imaging OR MRI OR magnetic resonance tomography OR nuclear magnetic resonance OR NMR	436,285
2	Positron emission tomography OR PET	48,019
3	Bone OR Skeletal OR Marrow	926,376
4	Step 1 AND 2 AND 3	704

cutaneous melanoma in 35 patients. All examinations were performed within a 24- to 72-hour time interval. Whole-body MRI and ^{18}F-FDG–PET/CT data sets were evaluated by different observers who were blinded to the findings of the other imaging modality. Histopathologic results, imaging, or clinical follow-up were used as the standard of reference, which indicated the presence of 14 bone marrow metastases in the studied population. Lesion-based sensitivity of whole-body MRI for the detection of bone marrow metastases was 82.8% and that of ^{18}F-FDG–PET/CT was 71.4%. Furthermore, whole-body DWI detected 2 additional bone marrow metastases that were not seen at gadolinium-enhanced T1-weighted and STIR whole-body MRI. One of the conclusions of the investigators was that whole-body MRI, including DWI, may be a more accurate method for the detection of bone marrow metastases. The small number of patients and bone marrow metastases in this study, however, precludes drawing a definitive conclusion. Furthermore, it is not clear how many bone marrow metastases were histopathologically confirmed.[43]

Squillaci and colleagues[44] compared axial T1-weighted, T2-weighted, STIR, fat-saturated multiphase gadolinium-enhanced T1-weighted, and coronal gadolinium-enhanced T1-weighted whole-body MRI at 3.0T with ^{18}F-FDG–PET/CT for restaging of 20 consecutive patients with previously surgically treated colorectal carcinoma. Whole-body MRI was performed within 10 days after ^{18}F-FDG–PET/CT. Whole-body MRI and ^{18}F-FDG–PET/CT data sets were evaluated by different observers who were blinded to the findings of the other imaging modality. Histology or clinical follow-up of 3 to 6 months served as the standard of reference. Whole-body MRI and ^{18}F-FDG–PET/CT detected 9 bone marrow metastases in 3 patients. One spine lesion was missed at ^{18}F-FDG–PET/CT whereas 1 rib lesion was missed at whole-body MRI. Because of the small number of patients with bone marrow metastases, however, no conclusions can be drawn based on these results.[44]

Takano and colleagues[45] prospectively compared T1-weighted, T2-weighted, and axial diffusion-weighted whole-body MRI with ^{18}F-FDG–PET for the evaluation of metastatic disease in 11 patients with malignant pheochromocytoma or paraganglioma. Whole-body MRI and ^{18}F-FDG–PET were performed within 1 week. Whole-body MRI and ^{18}F-FDG–PET data sets were evaluated by different observers who were blinded to the findings of the other imaging modality. Whole-body MRI demonstrated 60 bone marrow metastases in 9 of 11 patients, of which 15 were not visualized at MRI. ^{18}F-FDG–PET demonstrated 49 bone marrow metastases in 9 of 11 patients, of which 4 were not visualized at ^{18}F-FDG–PET. Significant drawbacks of this study, however, are the low number of patients and the complete lack of a reference standard.[45]

Ribrag and colleagues[46] prospectively compared coronal T1-weighted and STIR whole-body MRI at 1.5T with ^{18}F-FDG–PET/CT for the detection of bone marrow involvement in 43 patients with newly diagnosed aggressive non-Hodgkin lymphoma. Whole-body MRI and ^{18}F-FDG–PET/CT were performed within 1 week. Whole-body MRI and ^{18}F-FDG–PET/CT data sets were evaluated by different observers who were blinded to the findings of the other imaging modality. Initial whole-body MRI and ^{18}F-FDG–PET/CT studies, follow-up whole-body MRI and ^{18}F-FDG–PET/CT studies, BMB, or bone marrow aspiration served as the standard of reference. According to the standard of reference, 9 of 43 patients had bone marrow involvement. Patient-based sensitivities of whole-body MRI and FDG–PET/CT for the detection of bone marrow involvement were 100%. Lesion-based sensitivities of whole-body MRI and FDG–PET/CT for the detection of bone marrow involvement were 83% and 96%. The investigators reported that patient-based and lesion-based sensitivities of both imaging modalities were similar. Because of the low number of patients with bone marrow metastases (of which only 2 were histopathologically confirmed), however, no conclusions can be drawn based on these results. Furthermore, initial whole-body MRI and ^{18}F-FDG–PET/CT studies formed part of the reference standard.[46]

Ohno and colleagues[32] prospectively compared the diagnostic performance of coronal and sagittal in-phase (non–contrast-enhanced and gadolinium-enhanced) T1-weighted, opposed-phase T1-weighted, and STIR whole-body MRI at 1.5T with ^{18}F-FDG–PET for M-stage assessment in 90 consecutive lung cancer patients before treatment. All studies were performed in random order within 3 weeks of diagnosis and before treatment. Whole-body MRI and ^{18}F-FDG–PET data sets were evaluated by different observers. The final M-stage and metastasis of a given site were determined based on the results of standard imaging; pathologic examinations from endoscopic, CT-guided, or surgical biopsies; and follow-up examinations for more than 20 months in every patient. According to the standard of reference, there were 25 bone metastases. Although the area under the receiver operating characteristic curve and sensitivity of whole-body MRI (0.93 and 88%, respectively) regarding the detection of bone metastases on a per-site basis were not significantly different ($P>.05$) from those of ^{18}F-FDG–PET (0.90 and 88%, respectively), specificity and accuracy of whole-body MRI (96.1% and 94.8%, respectively) were significantly higher ($P<.05$) than those of ^{18}F-FDG–PET (88.3% and 88.2%, respectively). The investigators stated that whole-body MRI constitutes a significantly specific and accurate screening tool for assessment of bone metastases and warrants being considered for adoption as the primary screening tool, or a complementary screening tool, for ^{18}F-FDG–PET assessment of bone metastases in lung cancer patients. Advanced whole-body MRI sequences, however, such as whole-body DWI were not acquired in this study, and ^{18}F-FDG–PET was performed using a stand-alone PET system, as a result of which diagnostic performances may have been underestimated. Furthermore, the total number of patients with bone metastatic disease was not specified, and histopathologic confirmation was not possible for every bone metastasis.[32]

Schmidt and colleagues[47] prospectively compared coronal T1-weighted and STIR whole-body MRI and sagittal T1-weighted and STIR MRI of the spine with full-dose, contrast-enhanced ^{18}F-FDG–PET/CT for the detection or follow-up of bone metastases in 30 consecutive patients with various malignancies (breast carcinoma, n = 13; gastrointestinal tract tumor, n = 7; cancer of unknown primary, n = 4; malignant melanoma,

n = 3; hepatocellular carcinoma, n = 1; non-Hodgkin lymphoma, n = 1; and rhabdomyosarcoma, n = 1). Whole-body MRI and ^{18}F-FDG–PET/CT were performed within a maximum of 14 days. Whole-body MRI and ^{18}F-FDG–PET/CT data sets were evaluated by different observers who were blinded to findings of the other imaging modality. All detected lesions at whole-body MRI and ^{18}F-FDG–PET/CT were cross-checked by radiologic follow-up studies (^{18}F-FDG–PET/CT, n = 10; CT, n = 8; bone scintigraphy, n = 7; conventional radiography, n = 5; MRI, n = 5; and whole-body MRI, n = 2) within at least 6 months as a standard of reference. According to the standard of reference, there were 102 bone metastases in 23 of 30 patients. In a patient-by-patient analysis, metastatic bone disease was revealed in all these 23 patients by whole-body MRI (sensitivity 100%) but was missed in 2 patients by ^{18}F-FDG–PET/CT (sensitivity 91%). Whole-body MRI falsely diagnosed metastatic bone disease in 1 patient that showed no evidence indicating bone malignancy in follow-up (specificity 80%) and was confirmed as focal red marrow. ^{18}F-FDG–PET/CT showed a specificity of 100%. Patient-based diagnostic accuracy was 96% for whole-body MRI and 93% for ^{18}F-FDG–PET/CT. In a region-by-region analysis, sensitivity and specificity of whole-body MRI were 94% and 76%. ^{18}F-FDG–PET/CT showed a sensitivity of 78% and specificity of 80%. Differences in sensitivity between both modalities were significant ($P<.001$); differences in specificity were not significant ($P<.05$). Diagnostic accuracy was 91% for whole-body MRI and 78% for [18]F-^{18}F-FDG–PET/CT; this difference was significant ($P<.05$). Large lesions with a diameter greater than 2 cm were correctly diagnosed in 100% with whole-body MRI and 93% with ^{18}F-FDG–PET/CT, medium-sized lesions of 1 to 2 cm in 91% and 70%, and small-sized lesions below 1 cm in 88% and 56%, respectively. Thirteen percent of bone metastases diagnosed by ^{18}F-FDG–PET/CT in this study were non–[18]F-FDG–avid and final diagnosis was made with the CT data alone. The investigators concluded that diagnostic accuracy of whole-body MRI for bone marrow screening is superior to that of ^{18}F-FDG–PET/CT. Limitations of this study are the heterogeneous patient population, the lack of histologic proof for the detected lesions, verification bias, and the absence of advanced whole-body MRI sequences, such as whole-body DWI.[47]

Pfannenberg and colleagues[48] prospectively compared coronal STIR whole-body MRI combined with axial or coronal (gadolinium-enhanced) T1-weighted, fat-saturated T2-weighted and fluid-attenuated inversion recovery MRI of the brain, thorax, abdomen, and pelvis at 1.5T with full-dose, contrast-enhanced ^{18}F-FDG–PET/CT for staging of 64 consecutive patients with cutaneous melanoma. Whole-body MRI and ^{18}F-FDG–PET/CT were performed within a 24- to 72-hour time interval. Whole-body MRI and ^{18}F-FDG–PET/CT data sets were evaluated by different observers who were blinded to findings of the other imaging modality. The standard of reference for suspicious lesions included histology after resection (n = 65); imaging follow-up by ^{18}F-FDG–PET/CT, CT, dedicated MRI, ultrasound, bone scintigraphy, or conventional radiography (n = 267); or clinical follow-up (n = 88). According to this reference standard, there were a total of 35 bone metastases. Lesion-based sensitivity, specificity, PPV, NPV, and accuracy of whole-body MRI for the detection of bone metastases were 100%, 73.3%, 89.7%, 100%, and 92.0%, and those of ^{18}F-FDG–PET/CT were 91.4%, 80.0%, 91.4%, 80.0%, and 88.0%, respectively, without any significant difference between imaging modalities. Unfortunately, the number of patients with bone metastatic disease was not specified. Other study limitations are verification bias and that histopathologic confirmation was not possible for every bone metastasis. Furthermore, advanced whole-body MRI sequences, such as whole-body DWI, were not performed.[48]

Eschmann and colleagues[49] retrospectively compared coronal T1-weighted and STIR whole-body MRI combined with axial T1-weighted and STIR MRI of the thorax at 1.5T with full-dose, contrast-enhanced ^{11}C-choline–PET/CT for staging 42 patients with untreated (n = 17) or previously treated (n = 25) prostate cancer. In 21 patients, additional axial T2-weighted MRI of the pelvis was performed. Median time interval between whole-body MRI and ^{11}C-choline–PET/CT data sets was 1 day (range, 0–12 days). Whole-body MRI and ^{11}C-choline–PET/CT data sets were evaluated by different observers who were blinded to findings of the other imaging modality. Histopathologic results, follow-up, and consensus reading combining all imaging modalities and clinical and laboratory findings available served as the standard of reference. According to the reference standard, there were 40 bone metastases in 6 of 42 patients. Lesion-based sensitivities of whole-body MRI and ^{11}C-choline–PET/CT were 88.6% and 84.1%, respectively. Major limitations of this study are its retrospective design, which may have introduced selection bias; the low number of patients with bone metastases; verification bias; that whole-body MRI and ^{11}C-choline–PET/CT findings formed part of the reference standard; and the absence

of advanced whole-body MRI sequences, such as whole-body DWI.[49]

SUMMARY

Whole-body MRI, comprising T1-weighted and fat-saturated T2-weighted or STIR sequences, is a clinically feasible technique for the detection of metastases throughout the entire bone marrow. Promising new techniques that may improve assessment of the bone marrow are whole-body DWI and whole-body MRI after administration of USPIOs. Whole-body DWI cannot be performed yet, however, on all MRI systems and is still a laborious and time-consuming process. Furthermore, the availability of USPIOs is currently limited. Studies of the comparison between whole-body MRI and PET are scarce and the majority of these studies suffer from several methodologic shortcomings. Future well-designed prospective studies are needed to assess the diagnostic performance and cost-effectiveness of whole-body MRI compared with PET.

REFERENCES

1. Jemal A, Siegel R, Ward E, et al. Cancer statistics, 2009. CA Cancer J Clin 2009;59(4):225–49.
2. Coleman RE. Clinical features of metastatic bone disease and risk of skeletal morbidity. Clin Cancer Res 2006;12(20 Pt 2):6243s–9s.
3. Vanel D, Husband JE, Padhani AR. Bone metastases. In: Husband JE, Reznek RH, editors. Imaging in oncology. 2nd edition. London: Taylor & Francis; 1998. p. 1041–58.
4. Kricun ME. Red-yellow marrow conversion: its effect on the location of some solitary bone lesions. Skeletal Radiol 1985;14(1):10–9.
5. Krishnamurthy GT, Tubis M, Hiss J, et al. Distribution pattern of metastatic bone disease. A need for total body skeletal image. JAMA 1977;237(23):2504–6.
6. Bain BJ. Morbidity associated with bone marrow aspiration and trephine biopsy—a review of UK data for 2004. Haematologica 2006;91(9):1293–4.
7. Wang J, Weiss LM, Chang KL, et al. Diagnostic utility of bilateral bone marrow examination: significance of morphologic and ancillary technique study in malignancy. Cancer 2002;94(5):1522–31.
8. Miller TT. Bone tumors and tumorlike conditions: analysis with conventional radiography. Radiology 2008;246(3):662–74.
9. Edelstyn GA, Gillespie PJ, Grebbell FS. The radiological demonstration of osseous metastases. Experimental observations. Clin Radiol 1967;18(2): 158–62.
10. Kröpil P, Fenk R, Fritz LB, et al. Comparison of whole-body 64-slice multidetector computed

tomography and conventional radiography in staging of multiple myeloma. Eur Radiol 2008; 18(1):51–8.

11. Mahnken AH, Wildberger JE, Gehbauer G, et al. Multidetector CT of the spine in multiple myeloma: comparison with MR imaging and radiography. AJR Am J Roentgenol 2002;178(6):1429–36.

12. Mettler FA Jr, Huda W, Yoshizumi TT, et al. Effective doses in radiology and diagnostic nuclear medicine: a catalog. Radiology 2008;248(1):254–63.

13. Liu FY, Chang JT, Wang HM, et al. [18F]fluorodeoxyglucose positron emission tomography is more sensitive than skeletal scintigraphy for detecting bone metastasis in endemic nasopharyngeal carcinoma at initial staging. J Clin Oncol 2006;24(4): 599–604.

14. Basu S, Alavi A. Bone marrow and not bone is the primary site for skeletal metastasis: critical role of [18F]fluorodeoxyglucose positron emission tomography in this setting. J Clin Oncol 2007;25(10):1297.

15. Vogler JB 3rd, Murphy WA. Bone marrow imaging. Radiology 1988;168(3):679–93.

16. Vande Berg BC, Malghem J, Lecouvet FE, et al. Magnetic resonance imaging of normal bone marrow. Eur Radiol 1998;8(8):1327–34.

17. Basu S, Torigian D, Alavi A. Evolving concept of imaging bone marrow metastasis in the twenty-first century: critical role of FDG-PET. Eur J Nucl Med Mol Imaging 2008;35(3):465–71.

18. Even-Sapir E. Imaging of malignant bone involvement by morphologic, scintigraphic, and hybrid modalities. J Nucl Med 2005;46(8):1356–67.

19. Mirowitz SA, Apicella P, Reinus WR, et al. MR imaging of bone marrow lesions: relative conspicuousness on T1-weighted, fat-suppressed T2-weighted, and STIR images. AJR Am J Roentgenol 1994;162(1):215–21.

20. Yasumoto M, Nonomura Y, Yoshimura R, et al. MR detection of iliac bone marrow involvement by malignant lymphoma with various MR sequences including diffusion-weighted echo-planar imaging. Skeletal Radiol 2002;31(5):263–9.

21. Hanna SL, Fletcher BD, Fairclough DL, et al. Magnetic resonance imaging of disseminated bone marrow disease in patients treated for malignancy. Skeletal Radiol 1991;20(2):79–84.

22. Schweitzer ME, Levine C, Mitchell DG, et al. Bull's-eyes and halos: useful MR discriminators of osseous metastases. Radiology 1993;188(1):249–52.

23. Mahnken AH, Wildberger JE, Adam G, et al. Is there a need for contrast-enhanced T1-weighted MRI of the spine after inconspicuous short tau inversion recovery imaging? Eur Radiol 2005; 15(7):1387–92.

24. Tokuda O, Hayashi N, Matsunaga N. MRI of bone tumors: fast STIR imaging as a substitute for T1-weighted contrast-enhanced fat-suppressed spin-echo imaging. J Magn Reson Imaging 2004; 19(4):475–81.

25. Takahara T, Imai Y, Yamashita T, et al. Diffusion weighted whole body imaging with background body signal suppression (DWIBS): technical improvement using free breathing, STIR and high resolution 3D display. Radiat Med 2004; 22(4):275–82.

26. Nakanishi K, Kobayashi M, Nakaguchi K, et al. Whole-body MRI for detecting metastatic bone tumor: diagnostic value of diffusion-weighted images. Magn Reson Med Sci 2007;6(3):147–55.

27. Takenaka D, Ohno Y, Matsumoto K, et al. Detection of bone metastases in non-small cell lung cancer patients: comparison of whole-body diffusion-weighted imaging (DWI), whole-body MR imaging without and with DWI, whole-body FDG-PET/CT, and bone scintigraphy. J Magn Reson Imaging 2009;30(2):298–308.

28. Hackländer T, Scharwächter C, Golz R, et al. [Value of diffusion-weighted imaging for diagnosing vertebral metastases due to prostate cancer in comparison to other primary tumors]. Rofo 2006;178(4): 416–24 [in German].

29. Kwee TC, Takahara T, Ochiai R, et al. Diffusion-weighted whole-body imaging with background body signal suppression (DWIBS): features and potential applications in oncology. Eur Radiol 2008; 18(9):1937–52.

30. Lauenstein TC, Freudenberg LS, Goehde SC, et al. Whole-body MRI using a rolling table platform for the detection of bone metastases. Eur Radiol 2002; 12(8):2091–9.

31. Ghanem N, Kelly T, Altehoefer C, et al. [Whole-body MRI in comparison to skeletal scintigraphy for detection of skeletal metastases in patients with solid tumors]. Radiologe 2004;44(9):864–73 [in German].

32. Ohno Y, Koyama H, Nogami M, et al. Whole-body MR imaging vs. FDG-PET: comparison of accuracy of M-stage diagnosis for lung cancer patients. J Magn Reson Imaging 2007;26(3):498–509.

33. Lee KC, Sud S, Meyer CR, et al. An imaging biomarker of early treatment response in prostate cancer that has metastasized to the bone. Cancer Res 2007;67(8):3524–8.

34. Lee KC, Bradley DA, Hussain M, et al. A feasibility study evaluating the functional diffusion map as a predictive imaging biomarker for detection of treatment response in a patient with metastatic prostate cancer to the bone. Neoplasia 2007;9(12): 1003–11.

35. Jaffe CC. Measures of response: RECIST, WHO, and new alternatives. J Clin Oncol 2006;24(20):3245–51.

36. Sénéterre E, Weissleder R, Jaramillo D, et al. Bone marrow: ultrasmall superparamagnetic iron oxide for MR imaging. Radiology 1991;179(2):529–33.

37. Vande Berg BC, Lecouvet FE, Kanku JP, et al. Ferumoxides-enhanced quantitative magnetic resonance imaging of the normal and abnormal bone marrow: preliminary assessment. J Magn Reson Imaging 1999;9(2):322–8.

38. Daldrup-Link HE, Rummeny EJ, Ihssen B, et al. Iron-oxide-enhanced MR imaging of bone marrow in patients with non-Hodgkin's lymphoma: differentiation between tumor infiltration and hypercellular bone marrow. Eur Radiol 2002;12(6):1557–66.

39. Metz S, Lohr S, Settles M, et al. Ferumoxtran-10-enhanced MR imaging of the bone marrow before and after conditioning therapy in patients with non-Hodgkin lymphomas. Eur Radiol 2006;16(3):598–607.

40. Hargaden G, O'Connell M, Kavanagh E, et al. Current concepts in whole-body imaging using turbo short tau inversion recovery MR imaging. AJR Am J Roentgenol 2003;180(1):247–52.

41. Takahara T, Kwee TC, Kifune S, et al. Whole-body MRI using a sliding table and repositioning surface coil approach. Eur Radiol 2009. DOI:10.1007/s00330-009-1674-1.

42. Heusner T, Gölitz P, Hamami M, et al. "One-stop-shop" staging: should we prefer FDG-PET/CT or MRI for the detection of bone metastases? Eur J Radiol 2009. DOI:10.1016/j.ejrad.2009.10.031.

43. Laurent V, Trausch G, Bruot O, et al. Comparative study of two whole-body imaging techniques in the case of melanoma metastases: advantages of multi-contrast MRI examination including a diffusion-weighted sequence in comparison with PET-CT. Eur J Radiol 2009. DOI:10.1016/j.ejrad.2009.04.059.

44. Squillaci E, Manenti G, Mancino S, et al. Staging of colon cancer: whole-body MRI vs. whole-body PET-CT–initial clinical experience. Abdom Imaging 2008;33(6):676–88.

45. Takano A, Oriuchi N, Tsushima Y, et al. Detection of metastatic lesions from malignant pheochromocytoma and paraganglioma with diffusion-weighted magnetic resonance imaging: comparison with 18F-FDG positron emission tomography and 123I-MIBG scintigraphy. Ann Nucl Med 2008;22(5):395–401.

46. Ribrag V, Vanel D, Leboulleux S, et al. Prospective study of bone marrow infiltration in aggressive lymphoma by three independent methods: whole-body MRI, PET/CT and bone marrow biopsy. Eur J Radiol 2008;66(2):325–31.

47. Schmidt GP, Schoenberg SO, Schmid R, et al. Screening for bone metastases: whole-body MRI using a 32-channel system versus dual-modality PET-CT. Eur Radiol 2007;17(4):939–49.

48. Pfannenberg C, Aschoff P, Schanz S, et al. Prospective comparison of 18F fluorodeoxyglucose positron emission tomography/computed tomography and whole-body magnetic resonance imaging in staging of advanced malignant melanoma. Eur J Cancer 2007;43(3):557–64.

49. Eschmann SM, Pfannenberg AC, Rieger A, et al. Comparison of 11C-choline-PET/CT and whole body-MRI for staging of prostate cancer. Nuklearmedizin 2007;46(5):161–8.

Assessment of Response to Therapy for Bone Metastases: Is it Still a Challenge in Oncology?

J. Collignon, MD[a],*, C. Gennigens, MD[a],
G. Jerusalem, MD, PhD[a,b]

KEYWORDS

• Bone metastasis • Response assessment • Breast cancer
• Prostate cancer • Diagnostic imaging • FDG-PET

Bone is a common site of tumor metastases. Most patients with bone metastases present with pain at the time of diagnosis. Bone is the most common site of metastases in breast cancer. It is the first site of disease dissemination in 25% to 50% of all patients developing metastases from breast cancer.[1] About 70% of patients dying from breast and prostate cancers have evidence of bone metastases. Autopsy data also reveal a 40% incidence of bone metastases at the time of death in thyroid, kidney, lung, and pancreas carcinoma.

Bone metastases have a major effect on quality of life, in particular by impairing the motility of the patient. Pain, hypercalcemia, pathologic fracture, and spinal cord compression are the most important complications. Spinal cord compression is considered an emergency clinical situation that requires neurosurgical intervention or radiotherapy.

Patients with bone-only disease have a better prognosis than patients with visceral disease. In lung cancer, for example, the median overall survival is 13 to 25 months for bone-only disease, compared with 6 to 7 months in patients with visceral metastases. Survival also depends on the tumor type: a better prognosis is observed in breast cancer or prostate cancer. Long-term survival, up to several years, is frequently observed. The type of bone lesion is also an important factor. The prognosis is much better for sclerotic lesions compared with lytic lesions.

Accurate response evaluation is important in oncology. Most of the anticancer treatments, in particular chemotherapy, are highly toxic, but only a fraction of all patients respond to them. There is an unmet need for response evaluation in bone metastases in the routine practice of oncology as well as in the context of a clinical trial.

Measuring tumor shrinkage on CT based on Response Evaluation Criteria in Solid Tumors (RECIST) criteria represents the current standard in response evaluation in oncology. However, bone metastases are considered unmeasurable lesions. In the past, most clinical trials excluded patients with bone-only metastases. In routine practice, assessment of response is based more on the oncologist's own experience than on published criteria. Many treatments used in this patient population are only validated in patients presenting with visceral metastases.

There is also a specific need for response evaluation when targeted treatments are used. The new antiangiogenic therapies and other targeted therapies are generally not cytotoxic but

[a] Division of Medical Oncology, Domaine Universitaire, B35, CHU Sart Tilman Liège, Belgium
[b] University of Liège, Domaine Universitaire, B35, Liege 4000, Belgium
* Corresponding author.
E-mail address: Joelle.collignon@chu.ulg.ac.be

PET Clin 5 (2010) 311–326
doi:10.1016/j.cpet.2010.05.002

cytostatic, and produce disease stabilization rather than tumor regression. Evaluation of the tumor size is not useful. Imaging techniques are now required to monitor biologic phenomena such as tumor angiogenesis. Functional imaging techniques are the most appropriate methods for response assessment in these situations.

BIOLOGY AND MECHANISM OF BONE METASTASES

The most common metastatic sites are spine, pelvis, ribs, skull, and proximal long bones. Metastases may reach the skeleton by direct invasion from the primary tumor or by dissemination from a secondary site. Hematogenous spread is more frequent than lymphatic spread or direct invasion. The venous route, especially Batson paravertebral plexus, seems to be more important than the arterial route. The distribution of Batson venous plexus, as well as the overall skeletal vascularity, results in a predilection for hematogenous spread to the axial skeleton and the proximal long bones.[2] Metastases to the peripheral bones of the extremities are rare. The vertebrae and pelvis (**Fig. 1**) are the most frequent sites of bone metastases, followed by ribs, skull, and femur; this is true in breast and prostate cancers. The cells infiltrate first the medullar cavity before they develop an extension to the cortex. Eighty percent of bone metastases involve the red marrow rich axial skeleton.

Bone metastases have different patterns of presentation. Some lesions are purely or mostly destructive (osteolytic) with extensive bone destruction and no bone formation, such as is observed in myeloma, lung or renal cell carcinoma, and sometimes in breast cancer. Others are mostly bone forming (osteoblastic), as is frequently the case for metastases from prostate cancer or hormonosensitive breast cancer. However, osteolytic and osteoblastic lesions are 2 extremes and, in most patients, bone metastases have a combination of both elements.[3] Some studies suggest that, in prostate cancer, prostate-specific antigen (PSA) can have a crucial role in the formation of osteoblastic bone metastases by promoting osteoblastic proliferation and apoptosis of osteoclast precursors.[4] Nevertheless, not all prostate bone metastases are osteoblastic: up to 30% of bone metastases from prostate cancer are osteolytic or mixed lesions.[2]

Bone destruction is a late event in the development of bone metastases. Tumor cell proliferation in the bone is the first event. A local reaction is later observed against these tumor cells and results in activation of osteoclasts or osteoblasts.

These different steps and interactions are better understood at the molecular level. This knowledge has led to the development of specific drugs and targeted therapies in the treatment and the prevention of bone metastasis. A consensus in this field was reported by the Second Cambridge Conference in 2008.[5] Evaluation of the efficacy of these treatments is an important clinical challenge.

The best imaging modality is not necessarily the same in all patients. It may depend on the treatment modality because each imaging technique gives specific information, such as tissue density, tumor metabolism, water content, or tumor vascularization.

HOW TO EVALUATE THE BONE RESPONSE

Clinical evaluation of cancer treatment effects needs to assess the change in tumor burden. Objective response (tumor shrinkage) and the time to disease progression are important end points in clinical trials (**Table 1**). This information is also used in the routine practice of clinical oncology for treatment decisions.

Since the late 1970s, several classification systems have been developed to report the treatment effect. Classifications developed 30 years ago defined response based on size criteria on

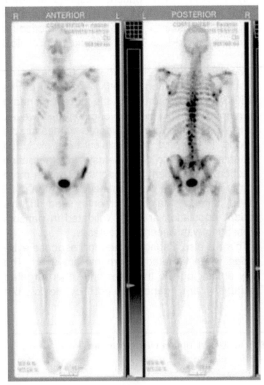

Fig. 1. Bone scan from a cancer patient showing usual distribution of bone metastases on axial skeleton.

Table 1
Response definition in clinical trial

Response Criteria	Definition
Pathologic complete response	No residual tumor on histopathologic analysis
Complete response (CR)	No residual lesion
Partial response (PR)	Decrease in size of measurable lesion
Stable disease	No change or minimum change in diameter of tumor
Progressive disease (PD)	Increase in size or new lesions

planar radiography. Despite the enormous progress in medical imaging, the definition of response is still mainly based on size criteria. Only recently has information from functional imaging techniques, such as 2-[^{18}F]fluoro-2-deoxy-D-glucose (FDG)-PET, been integrated into the classification systems.

International Union Against Cancer and World Health Organization Classifications

The first classifications, by the International Union Against Cancer (Union Internationale Contre Le Cancer, UICC) and the World Health Organization (WHO), were based on results from conventional radiographs (XR) and skeletal scintigraphy (SS);

they used the change in the summing of the products of bidimensional measurements of target lesions before and after treatment. They classified the patients into 4 response groups: complete response (CR), partial response (PR), stable disease, and progressive disease (PD). These measures can be used for bone assessment (**Table 2**).

Limitations

1. Low sensitivity of bone radiograph at diagnosis (many known bone lesions are false-negative)
2. Bone turnover is slow and it can take several months to show changes when such criteria

Table 2
Criteria for definition of bone response: useful classification

Response Type	UIAC	WHO
CR	Disappearance of all known disease Lytic lesions should have radiologic evidence of calcification	Complete disappearance of all lesions on radiograph or scan for at least 4 wk
PR	At least 50% decrease in size of measurable lesions No new lesions or progressive lesions	Partial decrease in size of lytic lesions, recalcification of lytic lesions, or decreased density of blastic lesions for at least 4 wk
Stable disease	Unchanged, or between 25% increase and 50% decrease in size of measurable lesions	Because of the slow response of bone lesions, the classification of nonchange should not be applied until at least 8 wk after start of therapy
PD	New lesions appear There is a 25% or more increase in the sum of the products of the diameters of each lesion measured, except that, if an increase of less than 25% makes additional treatment necessary, this is also regarded as progression Mixed: some lesions persist whereas others progress, or new lesions appear Failure: some or all lesions progress or new lesions appear No lesions regress	Increase in size of existent lesions or appearance of new lesions

are used; there is a need for early response evaluation

3. Comparative measures on radiograph are difficult in daily practice.

RECIST Criteria

In 2000, the RECIST criteria were published.[6] The evaluation of bidimensional diameters was replaced by unidimensional measures of the largest diameter of target lesions. They also gave definitions of minimum size of measurable lesions and instructions on the number of lesions to follow (up to 10, a maximum of 5 per organ site).

Limitations

1. Definition of bone lesions as nonmeasurable lesions
2. Patients with bone-only metastases are excluded when measurable lesions are mandatory for participation in a clinical trial.

RECIST 1.1 Criteria

The new RECIST 1.1 criteria were developed to improve response evaluation. The new RECIST criteria define bone lesions as being measurable in certain conditions[1] as listed in the original report (**Table 3**):

1. Bone scintigraphy, PET scan, or plain films are not considered adequate imaging techniques to measure bone lesions. However, these techniques can be used to confirm the presence or disappearance of bone lesions.
2. Lytic bone lesions or mixed lytic-blastic lesions, with identifiable soft-tissue components, that can be evaluated by cross-sectional imaging techniques such as CT or MR imaging can be considered as measurable lesions if the soft-tissue component meets the definition of measurability as recommended (measurable

in at least 1 dimension with a minimum size of 10 mm).

3. Blastic bone lesions are nonmeasurable.

RECIST 1.1 gives also information on the definition of new lesions that should be unequivocal and not related to the use of different imaging techniques. In particular, attention must be paid to differences in scanning techniques, changes in imaging modality or healing, or flare-up phenomenon in preexisting lesions.

Limitations

1. The assessment of response in lesions previously treated by radiotherapy to decrease pain. Such lesions are usually considered nonmeasurable unless there was a tumor progression after radiotherapy.
2. Osteoblatic bone lesions are still nonmeasurable.
3. Response assessment in absence of size reduction because this is seen frequently with some new targeted therapies that only decrease the metabolic activity of these lesions.

MD Anderson Cancer Center Imaging Algorithm in Breast Cancer

In 2004, Hamaoka and colleagues[7] published 2 algorithms: 1 to be used for the diagnosis of bone metastases from breast cancer and 1 to be used in the assessment of bone response to treatment.

They used radiographs, bone scintigraphy, CT, and MR imaging for diagnosis and response evaluation. CT or MR imaging should be repeated every 2 to 6 months when used for response evaluation. CT and MR imaging can show bone response as early as 2 months after the beginning of treatment. The modality that gave the best evaluation of the lesion at diagnosis must be used to assess treatment response. The best technique is not the same

Table 3
RECIST 1.1 and bone lesions based on CT and MR imaging measure

CR	Disappearance of all target lesions
PR	30% decrease in the sum of diameters of target lesions, taking as reference the baseline sum diameters
PD	At least 20% increase in the sum of diameters of target lesions, taking as reference the smallest sum on study Appearance of new lesion on bone scan should be unequivocal: be aware of flare of preexisting lesion
SD	Neither sufficient shrinkage to qualify for PR nor sufficient increase to qualify for PD, taking as reference the smallest sum diameters while on study

Measurable lesion if soft tissue component by CT scan or MR imaging. PET can be used for appearance or disappearance of lesions. Blastic lesion are nonmeasurable.

for every patient, but depends on the type of tumor and the site of bone metastases.

In the MD Anderson response criteria, the result of assessment of bone response using CT or MR imaging is added to the UICC and WHO response criteria (**Table 4**).

These criteria were used in a retrospective study in 41 breast cancer patients. They compared MD Anderson response criteria with WHO classification for assessing bone response. Correlated with progression-free and overall survival, the response classification based on MD Anderson criteria was superior to the WHO classification for identifying responders and nonresponders.[8]

Limitations
1. Further studies are indicated to validate this classification prospectively in cohorts of patients with bone metastases.

Perspectives in Response Evaluation

The next step is to integrate functional imaging, such as PET and dynamic contrast-enhanced (DCE)-MR imaging, with the current modalities for response assessment.

All these classifications rely solely on imaging techniques. In clinical practice, other modalities of response evaluation should also be considered. The evolution of clinical symptoms, in particular pain, biochemical markers of bone turnover such as N-telopeptide cross-links of type 1 collagen[9,10] and tumor marker measurements such as PSA in prostate cancer[11] or CA 15.3 in breast cancer, can provide useful information.

When is Biopsy Needed?

CT-guided percutaneous needle biopsies of bone metastases are performed in many centers. However, in most patients a biopsy is not necessary. A history of cancer, clinical symptoms such as pain, tumor markers, or results from imaging studies, including the number and the localization of the lesions, may indicate a primary tumor at the origin of metastatic disease.

However, in some situations a histologic confirmation is mandatory:

1. Whenever there is any doubt about the diagnosis of metastatic disease. Solitary bone lesions can represent diagnostic difficulties. Imaging techniques and FDG-PET are particularly helpful in distinguishing between benign and malignant lesions. However, only tissue sampling is able to provide a definitive diagnosis.
2. A vertebral fracture needing surgery if the preoperative work-up suspects a nonosteoporotic cause in a patient without a history of cancer.[12] Imaging-guided percutaneous biopsy is a reliable method for histologic analysis, but

Table 4
MD Anderson: revised criteria proposed for assessment of bone response

Response Type	Criteria
CR	Complete fill-in or sclerosis of lytic lesion on XR and CT Disappearance of hot spots or tumor signal on SS, CT, or MR imaging Normalization of osteoblastic lesion on XR and CT
PR[a]	Sclerotic rim about initially lytic lesion or sclerosis of previously undetected lesion on XR or CT Partial fill-in or sclerosis of lytic lesion on XR or CT Regression of measurable lesion on XR, CT, or MR imaging Regression of lesion on SS (exclude rapid regression[b]) Decrease in blastic lesion on XR or CT
No change (stable disease)	No change in measurable lesion on XR, CT, or MR imaging No change in blastic lesion on XR, CT, or MR imaging No new lesion on XR, SS, CT, or MR imaging
PD	Increase in size of any existing measurable lesions on XR, SS (exclude flares), CT, or MR imaging Increase in activity on SS (exclude flares) or blastic/lytic lesion on XR or CT

[a] Every lesion need not have regressed to qualify for response, but no lesion should have progressed.
[b] Rapid osteolytic progression may show decreased osteoblastic activity, resulting in apparent regression on SS.

Adapted from Hamaoka T, Costelloe CM, Madewell JE, et al. Tumour response interpretation with new tumour response criteria vs the World Health Organisation criteria in patients with bone-only metastatic breast cancer. Br J Cancer 2010;102:651–7; with permission.

this is not the best diagnostic procedure when lesions are purely intraosseous. In this situation, primary open biopsy is mandatory.[13]

3. Unknown primary cancer presenting as bone metastases. Twenty-five percent of all patients suffering from an unknown primary tumor have bone metastases. When the metastases are limited to the skeleton, a bone biopsy is mandatory to determine the histology of the tumor. In a large Dutch population-based study published in 2002, 8% of all the patients presented with bone metastases as the only site of disease.[14]

4. Bone lesions in patients suffering from a primary that rarely produce bone metastases. A second primary tumor at the origin of these bone metastases should be excluded.

5. Bone metastases in a patient with an excellent prognosis or a relapse that occurs unexpectedly late in the course of the disease. Another primary at the origin of bone metastases should be excluded.

6. Biopsy could be important not only for the confirmation of metastatic disease but also to obtain new information concerning targets for anticancer treatment. For example, when breast cancer relapses, the clinician sometimes needs a biopsy to see whether tumor characteristics have changed. The presence or absence of hormone receptors will help to decide which treatment should be administered. Her-2 overexpression will also be evaluated.

WHICH TECHNIQUES ARE USEFUL?

It is important to know which imaging procedure is preferable in each situation. In clinical studies, the method is generally defined by the study protocol. RECIST 1.1 are used with increasing frequency and permit the assessment of bone lesions, with some limitations. Outside a clinical trial, RECIST 1.1 can also be used, but additional information is also provided by functional imaging techniques, and we try in our center to integrate information obtained by functional imaging techniques in the overall response evaluation of our patients.

XR

In UICC and WHO classifications, evaluation of response was by XR and SS. Because of their many limitations, they are no longer recommended for routine clinical care. To be visible on radiograph, the bone destruction must be extensive, with a loss of more than 50% of bone mineral content.

Limitations

1. The bone lesion will not appear on XR before several months.
2. Because of the time needed to see modifications, early diagnosis and assessment of bone response are difficult.

In daily practice, we frequently have patients with suspected bone lesions and normal radiograph findings. Negative radiograph studies in the presence of a positive bone scan do not rule out metastatic disease. If the radiograph is negative, further studies should be performed to formally exclude or confirm a bone relapse. However, standard radiograph studies of the bone remain useful to evaluate the risk of pathologic fractures because prophylactic surgery may be indicated.

Planar Bone Scintigraphy

Since its introduction in 1971, this has become the most commonly used technique for the screening of bone metastasis. It can give useful information on the localization of bone metastasis when recurrent disease is suspected. It allows a whole-body examination. Despite some limitations in sensitivity and specificity, it can give useful information for the localization of bone metastases. It is useful for response evaluation[15] but it cannot easily be used for early response evaluation because of the possible flare-up phenomenon. It visualizes the increase in osteoblastic activity and skeletal vascularity.

Limitations

1. This technique has limited resolution and cannot help the clinician in the evaluation of soft tissue adjacent to a bone lesion.
2. It can lead to many false-positive results in the case of degenerative disease, Paget disease, fracture, and inflammatory changes, especially in the elderly. The experience of the reader can reduce these problems, and clinical data also help in the interpretation of the bone scan.
3. False-negative results are common in osteolytic lesions and in rapidly growing bone metastases with no osteoblastic reaction.
4. The flare-up phenomenon (ie, increased osteoblastic activity as a consequence of new bone formation and bone reparative changes in the case of a successful treatment) has to be interpreted as a favorable response to treatment and not as a PD. In such cases, radiographs and CT will show increased sclerosis in previously osteolytic or mixed bone lesions.

Clinicians can also use clinical and biologic markers, such as bone pain, tumor markers, and bone resorption markers, for response evaluation.[16,17] If there is a response to therapy, the bone scan can remain positive for a long time. In the first months, new lesions can be observed that represent the healing of lesions too small to be detectable on the initial bone scintigraphy. A flare response usually lasts about 6 months after therapy and can be associated with a good prognosis in prostate cancer.[18] In breast cancer, the flare response is also well known.[19] This phenomenon is frequently observed and is associated with response to systemic therapy including hormonal treatment. Consequently, the oncologist has to be careful in interpreting bone scans performed in the first months after change of therapy because this flare phenomenon cannot be distinguished from PD.

As mentioned earlier, bone scan is used to establish CR or PD in the RECIST1.1 criteria but measurements are not possible.

Single-photon Emission Computed Tomography

Single-photon emission computed tomography (SPECT) is similar to bone scan but with tomographic imaging (**Fig. 4**D). It improves the accuracy of bone scans in areas such as the spine or the pelvis. Spine is the most common site for metastases from various tumors, and isolated spine metastases are observed in 20% to 50% of patients presenting with bone metastases. SPECT is more sensitive for skeletal metastases than planar bone scintigraphy because of better contrast and better visibility of deeply located lesions.[20]

CT and MR Imaging

CT is superior to XR in the diagnosis of skeletal metastases and should be performed when bone scintigraphy is positive and conventional examinations are normal.[21] CT confirms half of the sites that are positive on bone scan but negative on radiographs. It can also explain causes of false-positive bone scan results such as degenerative disease. In metastases, it helps in evaluating osseous destruction extension and the risk of fracture. It distinguishes osteolytic from osteoblastic lesions.

In some circumstances, CT can be more than an anatomic imaging technique because contrast enhancement and tissue density may also be used for response evaluation.

MR imaging adds useful information to CT results because MR imaging visualizes the bone marrow and is superior to the other techniques in the evaluation of the extraosseous growth of the metastases. MR imaging shows better diagnostic accuracy than CT scan for spinal metastases and is the gold standard for the evaluation of the spine.[20] MR imaging is useful for the definition of the target field of irradiation when radiotherapy is planned. Access to MR imaging is an important limitation in many countries, in particular if repeated evaluations are needed. Another limitation for MR imaging is that this technique is unable to distinguish between lytic and sclerotic lesions; a particularly important issue for evaluation of the risk of pathologic fractures.

MR imaging and CT scan are used in the evaluation of response with RECIST 1.1 and, more recently, by MD Anderson algorithms for the diagnosis and assessment of response. The most important limitation is that criteria for response are still based on size criteria without any metabolic evaluation. The use of CT and MR imaging in such classifications also needs experience and time to evaluate the evolution of target lesions in the bone.

The performance of CT, MR imaging, and PET for response assessment should be compared carefully in clinical studies. Many data have been published on the comparative value for detecting lesions, as reported in the articles by Cook, Costelloe and colleagues, and Kwee and colleagues elsewhere in this issue, but more studies are needed in the evaluation of response with functional assessment.

Functional Imaging Techniques

For the clinician, these techniques are potentially useful in daily practice. However, further studies and internationally accepted guidelines are needed before these techniques can routinely be used.

PET

[18F]Fluoride [18F]Fluoride is a nonspecific bone marker first described in 1962. Bone scan using 99mTc-labeled diphosphonates remains the imaging technique of choice for the screening of bone metastases, but modern PET scanners increase the resolution of bone imaging while reducing the scanning time, and [18F]fluoride is thus being reintroduced into the routine clinical care. The role of [18F]fluoride in prostate cancer has been shown in a recent review.[18] Some limitations are related to false-negative results in patients presenting highly dense sclerotic bone lesions. PET/CT is highly sensitive and may replace unconventional bone scan in the future. At this time, the technique has a role in the diagnostic of bone metastases, as reviewed

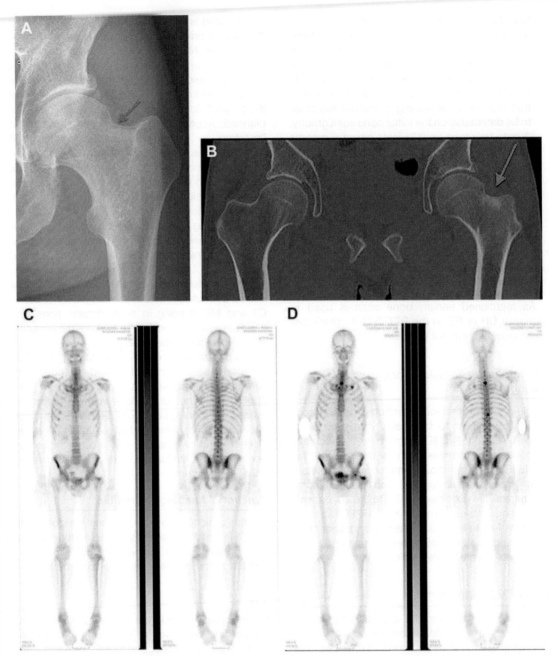

Fig. 2. Patient with metastatic gastrinoma and left hip pain. The radiograph was negative (*A*) and the CT scan (*B*) showed hip osteoblastic lesion that could be degenerative. Bone scan performed 6 months before suspected hip lesion (*C*) and a new bone scan performed because of hepatic relapse, clearly showed progressive bone disease (*D*).

in the article by Cook elsewhere in this issue. The role in response evaluation remains unknown.

FDG FDG, a glucose analogue, shows enhanced uptake in most malignant tumors. FDG-PET is used for diagnosis, staging, and detection of residual/recurrent cancer.[22] This technique evaluates tumor metabolism and consequently is potentially useful for the evaluation of response even before the observation of any change in size in responding tumors.

In bone metastases, the exact mechanism of FDG uptake is not fully understood, but it is probably directly taken up by the tumor tissue and not by the surrounding remodeled bone.[23]

Nuclear medicine imaging techniques can provide unique, biologically relevant, and prognostically important information that is unavailable through anatomic imaging.[24] PET as a functional imaging technology allows rapid and noninvasive in vivo assessment of several biologic processes targeted by anticancer therapies. The uptake of FDG is decreased in responding tumors. The standardized uptake value (SUV), also referred to as the differential uptake ratio and differential absorption ratio, has been widely used for tumor FDG uptake assessment.[22] Changes in SUV are useful for assessment of therapeutic effect. A decrease of 10% to 30% can be seen after 1 cycle in patients responding to chemotherapy. Several studies have tried to monitor response and correlate the early metabolic response with time to progression and survival in lymphoma[25,26] and in solid tumors.[27]

The modalities of patient preparation before performing a PET study are important for the performance of this imaging technique. Specific recommendations were reviewed by the European Organisation for Research and Treatment of Cancer (EORTC) PET group.[22] In clinical oncology, the role of PET response evaluation has steadily increased during the past year. However, the currently recommended criteria for assessment of response in bone metastases do not integrate PET information. Prospective studies are needed, although some data in favor of using PET for response evaluation are now available. A decrease in SUV shown by PET/CT has been positively correlated with response duration after therapy for bone metastases from breast cancer.[28] Another study correlated changes in serial FDG-PET with time to progression.[29] Changes in tumor metabolism evaluated by PET/CT occur more rapidly than the uptake of the radiotracer used for bone scanning and this could be a method for early assessment of response to chemotherapy or hormonal therapy.[20]

Studies evaluating the role of FDG-PET in the detection of bone metastases have given conflicting results, with sensitivity ranging from 56.5% to 100%.[30]

FDG-PET evaluation in bone metastases has distinct patterns in osteolytic and osteoblastic lesions. Sclerotic lesions may be negative, as observed in some patients suffering from prostate or breast cancer. It not known whether this reflects differences in the metabolic activity of various cancer cells or if the difference is to the result of fewer cancer cells in osteoblastic lesions.

As with bone scan, metabolic flare has been described with FDG-PET and should predict good response to hormonal treatment.[31,32]

Clinical flare reaction has been found in 5% to 20% of women with advanced estrogen receptor–positive breast cancer when the antitumoral treatment was started. Symptoms are generally observed within 7 to 10 days of the initiation of hormonal therapy. The clinical flare is associated with prolonged objective response. Metabolic flare was described in patients with objective tumor regression. More recently, similar case reports were published in patients with lung cancer treated with bevacizumab for bone metastases. Three patients had bone metabolic flare and, at the same time, a reduction in lung tumor FDG uptake.[33]

There is a proposal to integrate a classification based on anatomic data (WHO and RECIST) and a classification based on functional imaging (EORTC PET response criteria) into a combined classification, the PET Response Criteria in Solid Tumors (PERCIST) criteria.[34] This new classification needs further evaluation in clinical trials and should be adapted to bone lesions.

Hybrid imaging Technological evolution has led to the combining of various imaging techniques such as PET/CT, SPECT/CT, and, in the near future, PET/MR imaging. These combined techniques are complementary in the evaluation of response because CT and MR imaging reveal changes in bone structure and size, and PET assesses metabolic response in tumor cells. Most of the studies have been performed with PET/CT systems. Du and colleagues[35] reported a study on 25 patients with breast cancer with bone metastases who were evaluated by sequential half-body PET/CT. One-hundred and forty-six lesions were classified as osteolytic, osteoblastic, or mixed. After the baseline PET/CT evaluation, the patients received antitumoral treatment, including hormonal therapy, chemotherapy, and radiotherapy, alone or in combination. PET/CT was repeated at intervals between 2 and 9 months during a period of 23 months: 80.5% of osteolytic lesions, 52% of osteoblastic lesions, and 55% of mixed lesions became FDG negative. After treatment, 76.4% of FDG-avid lesions became FDG negative but most of them remained abnormal on CT with predominantly osteoblastic appearances, and most remained positive on bone scan. The investigators concluded that FDG-PET/CT hybrid images better reflect the tumor activity of bone metastases. Another study retrospectively evaluated 102 women with metastatic breast cancer with combined PET/CT. They analyzed the SUV and total lesion glycolysis to evaluate metabolic change. Univariate analysis revealed that the increase in attenuation and the decrease in SUV were potential predictors of longer response duration. Multivariate analysis revealed that an increase in the change in SUV was a significant predictor of response duration.[28]

Sequential FDG-PET/CT plays a role in the evaluation of response in bone metastases. Prospective trials are needed to confirm these data and to investigate other cancers.

DCE imaging techniques Angiogenesis is the process of new blood vessel growth and is a key pathway for tumor growth, invasion, and metastasis. This process also occurs in bone marrow where proliferating tumor cells have to develop their blood supply. Many antiangiogenic drugs have been developed. These drugs tend to be cytostatic, and response cannot be evaluated with conventional imaging techniques. There is an urgent need to develop and validate noninvasive techniques for imaging tumor vasculature to monitor tumor angiogenesis in vivo in a sensitive and specific way. DCE-MR imaging and CT can be used to measure the properties of tissue microvasculature. DCE-MR imaging has been used in early clinical trials evaluating several antiangiogenic and antivascular drugs to obtain pharmacodynamic information.[36,37] DCE-CT and DCE-MR imaging can be used for early assessment of treatment response in bone metastases by calculating the parameters associated with blood volume and vessel permeability. Early response after antiangiogenic therapy has been assessed by DCE-CT and DCE-MR imaging in experimental animal models of breast cancer bone metastases.[38] A treatment response can be shown as early as a few days, or even hours, after an antiangiogenic treatment. These techniques need further integration in clinical studies and their availability remains limited. There is also a need for standardization of the response assessment.

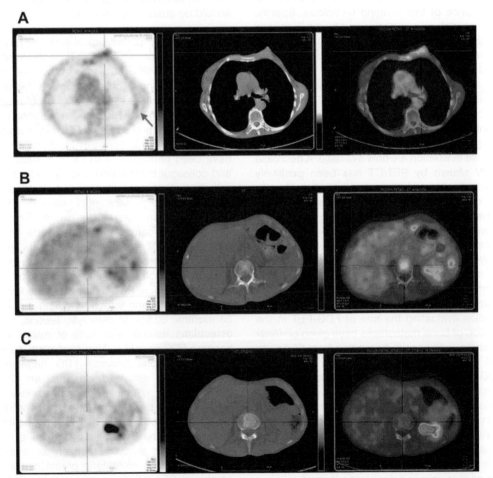

Fig. 3. Breast cancer with osteoblastic vertebral metastasis at diagnosis. FDG-PET was positive for the left breast (*A*) and the vertebral metastasis (*B*). In addition, a rib lesion was seen on FDG-PET only (*arrow*). After 7 months of hormonal therapy, there is no residual abnormal FDG uptake but there is no major change of the osteoblastic lesion on CT (*C*). The patient has a complete metabolic response.

APPLICABILITY FOR DAILY PRACTICE

There is a great deal of interest in defining a standard procedure for response evaluation in oncology within and outside a clinical trial. However, there is no universally accepted method for response evaluation in bone disease. For every technique, the experience of the reader is essential. In our daily practice, we frequently ask for the realization of several imaging procedures, conventional and functional imaging techniques, to best evaluate the treatment response. It is important to use the same imaging technique for diagnosis and for response evaluation. These studies should be done in the same technical conditions.

Clinical Case 1

Fig. 2 illustrates the difficulty in making a rapid diagnosis and in defining the best imaging procedure for response evaluation. This patient had a long history of metastatic gastrinoma in complete response after chemotherapy and hepatic graft. A bone scan (see **Fig. 2**C) shows femoral neck uptake 6 months before the patient developed bone pain. XR was normal and CT described an osteoblastic lesion caused by degenerative disease (see **Fig. 2**A,B). Because of a hepatic relapse, a new bone scan was performed. It indicated PD (see **Fig. 2**D). In such a case, only a multidisciplinary discussion including the oncologist and staff from the radiology and nuclear medicine department could determine the most appropriate staging, treatment, and response evaluation.

Clinical Case 2

Fig. 3A,B shows an osteoblastic bone metastasis in a patient with breast cancer. The patient received tamoxifen, an antitumoral hormonotherapy, for 3 months. Bone scan concluded at the time of

A

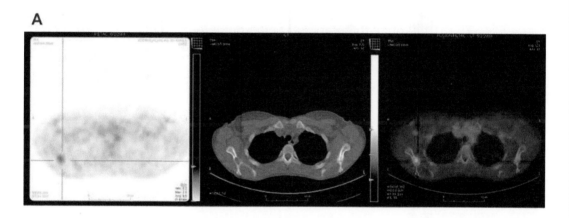

B

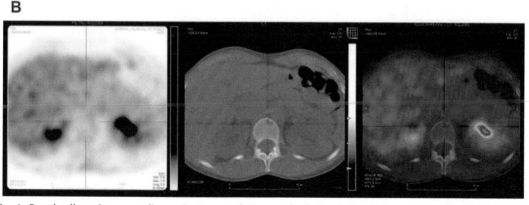

Fig. 4. Renal cell carcinoma at diagnosis. An osteolytic scapular lesion is clearly hypermetabolic (*A*) whereas an osteolytic vertebral metastasis does not take up FDG (*B*). The corresponding bone scan shows the lesions and the site of the cranial biopsy performed for pathologic diagnosis (*C*, planar images; *D*, SPECT). Bone scan was planned after 4 months of treatment with sunitinib. The scapular lesion remains stable whereas the L1 vertebral lesion has become a photopenic defect (*E*, planar images; *F*, SPECT). The scapular MR imaging was not modified after 4 months (*G*, T2 Fat Sat [FS]) and 8 months of treatment (*H*, T2 FS). Another bone scan, 2 months after stopping sunitinib, showed rapid PD (*I*).

reevaluation that the tumor progressed during treatment. Second-line hormonotherapy by letrozole, an aromatase inhibitor, was started. Reassessment of response by PET/CT was done after a further 4 months of treatment. PET/CT (see **Fig. 3**C) showed a good response, with the disappearance of all pathologic FDG uptakes in bone lesions and in the visceral metastases. However, anatomic evaluation by CT showed unchanged tumor extension. It is important to avoid misinterpretation, in particular early after starting anticancer treatment, because of the possible flare-up phenomenon. Clinicians should be aware of the limitations of the various imaging techniques

so that they are in a position to carefully select the most appropriate technique for each clinical situation. The results of these imaging techniques should always be interpreted in the context of the history of the patient, clinical symptoms (pain), and biochemical markers, including tumor markers.

Clinical Case 3

A young woman presented with a skull lesion. The primary work-up with PET/CT only showed 1 hypermetabolic bone lesion (see **Fig. 4**A) but CT also revealed a renal mass and another lytic

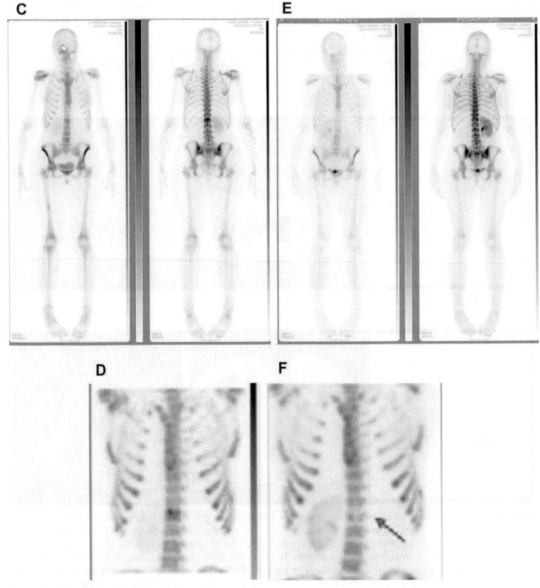

Fig. 4. (continued)

bone lesion without increased FDG uptake (see **Fig. 4**B). The nephrectomy revealed a renal carcinoma. Treatment with sunitinib, a multi tyrosine kinase inhibitor, was decided on as a first-line therapy. An evaluation of the treatment response performed by bone scan (see **Fig. 4**C,D) showed a metabolic response (see **Fig. 4**E,F) but only stable disease based on anatomic criteria by MR imaging (see **Fig. 4**G,H). The treatment was continued for more than a year until it had to be interrupted because of toxicity. A new bone scan after stopping sunitinib revealed rapid PD (see **Fig. 4**I).

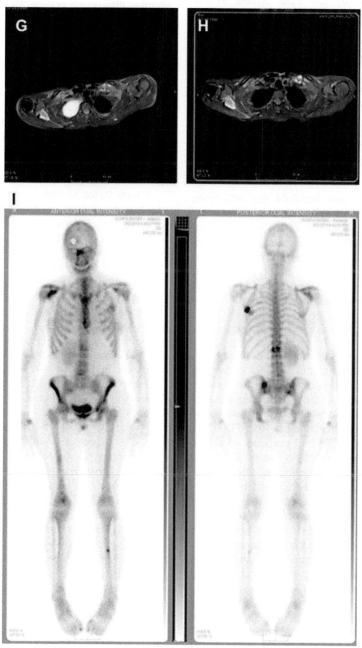

Fig. 4. (*continued*)

This clinical case highlights several key points concerning the use of imaging techniques in oncology:

1. CT should always be combined with FDG-PET for the work-up of bone metastases in patients with an unknown primary because some primary tumors can be FDG negative.
2. FDG-PET is not the imaging technique of choice for the diagnosis and staging of renal carcinoma. There are false-negative results caused by low FDG uptake in the tumor and urinary excretion of the radiotracer.[39] FDG-PET may add useful information concerning visceral metastases, lymph node infiltration, and metastatic bone disease.[40]
3. Bone lesions with different metabolic patterns and radiological appearances may coexist in a patient.
4. Functional imaging techniques should be considered when response to cytostatic drugs is evaluated, particularly in patients with bone metastases.

These clinical cases highlight the difficulties observed in routine clinical practice for evaluating bone disease. Response evaluation remains a major challenge. New functional response assessment criteria are needed, in particular for bone disease. A multidisciplinary discussion, taking into account all clinical and paraclinical results, should be organized to define the optimal treatment.

SUMMARY

Bone metastases are common and bone imaging is important for staging, but also for assessing the response. More and more data are contributing to new criteria for bone response assessment. In some conditions, RECIST 1.1 allows the evaluation of bone metastases, and FDG-PET has been introduced for that purpose. In breast cancer, MD Anderson criteria were developed with the combined use of radiograph, bone scan, CT, and MR imaging. FDG-PET and bone scan seem complementary because of their different sensitivities for detecting osteoblastic and osteolytic bone lesions. For FDG-PET, the advantages are that it is not limited to bone but allows assessment of primary tumor, lymph nodes, and visceral metastases in one imaging study, and it is also helpful in the assessment of response.

The criteria currently recommended for bone assessment should be improved. There is a need for prospective evaluation of FDG-PET, and particularly for PET-CT. The combination of functional and anatomic imaging techniques is the most promising approach to this problem. PERCIST criteria are the first attempt to integrate both types of imaging procedures. PERCIST criteria should be extended to bone response assessment.

Another perspective is the evaluation of new imaging techniques such as DCE-MR imaging, which evaluates tumor vasculature. This method of response evaluation should be particularly interesting for the evaluation of response to antiangiogenic drugs. DCE combined with CT or MR imaging also needs prospective evaluation.

REFERENCES

1. Eisenhauer EA, Therasse P, Bogaerts J, et al. New response evaluation criteria in solid tumours: revised RECIST guideline (version 1.1). Eur J Cancer 2009; 45:228–47.
2. Messiou C, Cook G, deSouza NM. Imaging metastatic bone disease from carcinoma of the prostate. Br J Cancer 2009;101:1225–32.
3. Mundy GR. Metastasis to bone: causes, consequences and therapeutic opportunities. Nat Rev Cancer 2002;2:584–93.
4. Goya M, Ishii G, Miyamoto S, et al. Prostate-specific antigen induces apoptosis of osteoclast precursors: potential role in osteoblastic bone metastases of prostate cancer. Prostate 2006;66:1573–84.
5. Coleman RE, Guise TA, Lipton A, et al. Advancing treatment for metastatic bone cancer: consensus recommendations from the Second Cambridge Conference. Clin Cancer Res 2008; 14:6387–95.
6. Hayward JL, Carbone PP, Heusen JC, et al. Assessment of response to therapy in advanced breast cancer. Br J Cancer 1977;35:292–8.
7. Hamaoka T, Madewell JE, Podoloff DA, et al. Bone imaging in metastatic breast cancer. J Clin Oncol 2004;22:2942–53.
8. Hamaoka T, Costelloe CM, Madewell JE, et al. Tumour response interpretation with new tumour response criteria vs the World Health Organisation criteria in patients with bone-only metastatic breast cancer. Br J Cancer 2010;102:651–7.
9. Vinholes J, Coleman R, Lacombe D, et al. Assessment of bone response to systemic therapy in an EORTC trial: preliminary experience with the use of collagen cross-link excretion. European Organization for Research and Treatment of Cancer. Br J Cancer 1999;80:221–8.
10. Blomqvist C, Risteli L, Risteli J, et al. Markers of type I collagen degradation and synthesis in the monitoring of treatment response in bone metastases from breast carcinoma. Br J Cancer 1996;73:1074–9.
11. Chen SS, Chen KK, Lin AT, et al. Correlation between pretreatment serum biochemical markers and

treatment outcome for prostatic cancer with bony metastasis. J Chin Med Assoc 2009;72:301–6.

12. Pneumaticos SG, Chatziioannou SN, Savvidou C, et al. Routine needle biopsy during vertebral augmentation procedures. Is it necessary? Eur Spine J 2010. [Epub ahead of print].

13. Datir A, Pechon P, Saifuddin A. Imaging-guided percutaneous biopsy of pathologic fractures: a retrospective analysis of 129 cases. AJR Am J Roentgenol 2009;193:504–8.

14. van de Wouw AJ, Janssen-Heijnen ML, Coebergh JW, et al. Epidemiology of unknown primary tumours; incidence and population-based survival of 1285 patients in southeast Netherlands, 1984–1992. Eur J Cancer 2002;38:409–13.

15. Rosenthal DI. Radiologic diagnosis of bone metastases. Cancer 1997;80:1595–607.

16. Koizumi M, Matsumoto S, Takahashi S, et al. Bone metabolic markers in the evaluation of bone scan flare phenomenon in bone metastases of breast cancer. Clin Nucl Med 1999;24:15–20.

17. Coombes RC, Dady P, Parsons C, et al. Assessment of response of bone metastases to systemic treatment in patients with breast cancer. Cancer 1983;52:610–4.

18. Beheshti M, Langsteger W, Fogelman I. Prostate cancer: role of SPECT and PET in imaging bone metastases. Semin Nucl Med 2009;39:396–407.

19. Janicek MJ, Hayes DF, Kaplan WD. Healing flare in skeletal metastases from breast cancer. Radiology 1994;192:201–4.

20. Elgazzar AH, Kazem N. Metastatic bone disease: evaluation by functional imaging in correlation with morphologic modalities. Gulf J Oncolog 2009; Jan(5):9–21.

21. Muindi J, Coombes RC, Golding S, et al. The role of computed tomography in the detection of bone metastases in breast cancer patients. Br J Radiol 1983;56:233–6.

22. Young H, Baum R, Cremerius U, et al. Measurement of clinical and subclinical tumour response using [18F]-fluorodeoxyglucose and positron emission tomography: review and 1999 EORTC recommendations. European Organization for Research and Treatment of Cancer (EORTC) PET Study Group. Eur J Cancer 1999;35:1773–82.

23. Schirrmeister H. Detection of bone metastases in breast cancer by positron emission tomography. Radiol Clin North Am 2007;45:669–76, vi.

24. Wahl RL, Jacene H, Kasamon Y, et al. From RECIST to PERCIST: evolving considerations for PET response criteria in solid tumors. J Nucl Med 2009; 50(Suppl 1):122S–50S.

25. Jerusalem G, Beguin Y, Fassotte MF, et al. Whole-body positron emission tomography using 18F-fluorodeoxyglucose for posttreatment evaluation in Hodgkin's disease and non-Hodgkin's lymphoma has higher diagnostic and prognostic value than classical computed tomography scan imaging. Blood 1999;94:429–33.

26. Jerusalem G, Beguin Y. The place of positron emission tomography imaging in the management of patients with malignant lymphoma. Haematologica 2006;91:442–4.

27. Couturier O, Jerusalem G, N'Guyen JM, et al. Sequential positron emission tomography using [18F]fluorodeoxyglucose for monitoring response to chemotherapy in metastatic breast cancer. Clin Cancer Res 2006;12:6437–43.

28. Tateishi U, Gamez C, Dawood S, et al. Bone metastases in patients with metastatic breast cancer: morphologic and metabolic monitoring of response to systemic therapy with integrated PET/CT. Radiology 2008;247:189–96.

29. Specht JM, Tam SL, Kurland BF, et al. Serial 2-[18F]fluoro-2-deoxy-D-glucose positron emission tomography (FDG-PET) to monitor treatment of bone-dominant metastatic breast cancer predicts time to progression (TTP). Breast Cancer Res Treat 2007;105:87–94.

30. Fogelman I, Cook G, Israel O, et al. Positron emission tomography and bone metastases. Semin Nucl Med 2005;35:135–42.

31. Dehdashti F, Flanagan FL, Mortimer JE, et al. Positron emission tomographic assessment of "metabolic flare" to predict response of metastatic breast cancer to antiestrogen therapy. Eur J Nucl Med 1999;26:51–6.

32. Mortimer JE, Dehdashti F, Siegel BA, et al. Metabolic flare: indicator of hormone responsiveness in advanced breast cancer. J Clin Oncol 2001;19:2797–803.

33. Krupitskaya Y, Eslamy HK, Nguyen DD, et al. Osteoblastic bone flare on F18-FDG PET in non-small cell lung cancer (NSCLC) patients receiving bevacizumab in addition to standard chemotherapy. J Thorac Oncol 2009;4:429–31.

34. Weber WA. Assessing tumor response to therapy. J Nucl Med 2009;50(Suppl 1):1S–10S.

35. Du Y, Cullum I, Illidge TM, et al. Fusion of metabolic function and morphology: sequential [18F]fluorodeoxyglucose positron-emission tomography/computed tomography studies yield new insights into the natural history of bone metastases in breast cancer. J Clin Oncol 2007;25:3440–7.

36. Berstein L, Maximov S, Gershfeld E, et al. Neoadjuvant therapy of endometrial cancer with the aromatase inhibitor letrozole: endocrine and clinical effects. Eur J Obstet Gynecol Reprod Biol 2002;105:161–5.

37. Lockhart AC, Rothenberg ML, Dupont J, et al. Phase I study of intravenous vascular endothelial growth factor trap, aflibercept, in patients with advanced solid tumors. J Clin Oncol 2010;28:207–14.

38. Bauerle T, Bartling S, Berger M, et al. Imaging anti-angiogenic treatment response with DCE-VCT, DCE-MRI and DWI in an animal model of breast cancer bone metastasis. Eur J Radiol 2010;73:280–7.

39. Wang X, Tangjitgamol S, Liu J, et al. Response of recurrent uterine high-grade malignant mixed mullerian tumor to letrozole. Int J Gynecol Cancer 2005;15:1243–8.

40. Bouchelouche K, Oehr P. Positron emission tomography and positron emission tomography/computerized tomography of urological malignancies: an update review. J Urol 2008;179:34–45.

^{18}F-FDG-PET and PET/CT for Evaluating Primary Bone Tumors

Erik Mittra, MD, PhD*, Andrei Iagaru, MD

KEYWORDS

- Fluorodeoxyglucose • Positron emission tomography
- Sarcoma • Malignant • Benign • Multiple myeloma

Bone tumors can be primary (originating in the bone) or metastatic. Primary tumors of bone can be subdivided into benign and malignant variants. The latter includes sarcomas originating from skeletal tissue itself, such as osteogenic sarcoma (osteosarcoma) and Ewing sarcoma.[1] Soft-tissue sarcomas are a distinct but related group and include chondrosarcoma, fibrosarcoma, malignant fibrous histiocytoma, and others.[2] Taken together, sarcomas are a heterogeneous group of tumors originating from mesenchymal tissues. Multiple myeloma is a hematologic cancer but often (90% of the time) presents with bony lesions.[3] Benign bone tumors are a varied group and include osteochondroma, enchondroma, osteoid osteoma, and fibrous dysplasia, among others.[4]

Bone sarcomas are rare and account for 0.2% of all primary cancers in adults and approximately 5% of childhood malignancies. Soft-tissue sarcomas are also uncommon, representing approximately 0.7% of adult malignancies. However, in children younger than 15 years they represent 6.5% of all cancers. According to the 2009 American Cancer Society estimates, approximately 12,130 new cases were expected in 2009, comprising soft-tissue tumors (10,660) and bone and joints tumors (1470). The estimated number of deaths in 2009 from these tumors is 5080, including 3820 from soft-tissue tumors and 1260 from bone and joints tumors.[5] Treatment generally includes a combination of surgery, radiation therapy, and chemotherapy.

Diagnostic imaging plays an important role in the evaluation of patients with primary tumors of bone. Clinical imaging can be subdivided into either anatomic (conventional) or functional (molecular) imaging. Anatomic imaging includes radiography, ultrasound, computed tomography (CT), and magnetic resonance (MR) imaging.[6] Functional imaging includes ^{99m}Tc-methyl diphosphonate (MDP) bone scintigraphy and ^{18}F-fluorodeoxyglucose (FDG) PET.[6–8] FDG-PET has an important role in the evaluation of patients with various malignancies, including sarcomas.[9,10] PET was initially used alone, but increasingly is used concurrently with CT.[11,12] FDG-PET and PET/CT facilitates detection of local recurrence and metastatic disease, guidance at biopsy sites, prediction and monitoring response to therapy, and assessment of prognosis.

This article reviews the role of FDG-PET and PET/CT in the evaluation of malignant primary bone tumors, focusing on osteosarcoma and Ewing sarcoma. The role of FDG-PET and PET/CT in multiple myeloma and benign primary bone tumors is also discussed. Soft-tissue sarcomas are a large and distinct topic, beyond the scope of this article.

MALIGNANT TUMORS
Osteosarcoma

Osteogenic sarcoma is the most common malignant primary bone tumor. The peak incidence is

Division of Nuclear Medicine, Department of Radiology, Stanford Hospital and Clinics, 300 Pasteur Drive, Room H0101, Stanford, CA 94305-8521, USA
* Corresponding author.
E-mail address: erik.mittra@stanford.edu

PET Clin 5 (2010) 327–339
doi:10.1016/j.cpet.2010.04.004
1556-8598/10/$ – see front matter © 2010 Elsevier Inc. All rights reserved.

in the second decade of life, with a second peak in the elderly, in which case it is usually associated with underlying pathology such as Paget disease, medullary infarct, or prior irradiation.[1] Osteosarcoma is histologically characterized by the presence of osteoid within the tumor, and has a predilection for the metaphyseal regions of long bones. Osteosarcoma most commonly affects the distal femur, followed by the proximal tibia, proximal femur, proximal humerus, and jaw.[1] Taken together, the knee accounts for 50% to 60% of cases.

Patients often present with ongoing (dull or aching) pain at the affected site, which may be worse at night or not associated with activity. Diagnosis ultimately requires a bone biopsy. Treatment typically involves neoadjuvant chemotherapy followed by surgical resection of the primary tumor. The latter is preferentially a limb-salvaging procedure, although amputation may be required. Resection is followed by additional chemotherapy.[1]

Staging is important for prognosis and selection of proper therapy. The American Joint Commission on Cancer (AJCC) system for staging osteosarcoma relies on the tumor size, nodal involvement, metastatic disease, and grade of the tumor. The surgical staging system (Enneking system) also relies on the grade of the tumor, as well as extent of the primary tumor and presence of metastasis, if any. In the latter system, low-grade, localized tumors are Stage I, high-grade, localized tumors are Stage II, and metastatic tumors (regardless of grade) are Stage III.[4,13]

Imaging plays an important role in the diagnosis, staging, and posttherapy evaluation of osteosarcoma. Radiography, MR imaging, CT, and bone scintigraphy are the modalities traditionally used in osteosarcoma.[6] FDG-PET or PET/CT has a limited role in the diagnosis of osteosarcoma, but does have important roles in grading, staging, prognostication, evaluation of therapeutic response, and detection of recurrent disease (Table 1).[14,15] Under the revised 2009 Medicare National Coverage Determinations, the initial evaluation (diagnosis and staging) is covered normally, while subsequent evaluations (restaging and response to therapy) are covered under the Coverage with Evidence Development (CED) category.

As already mentioned, grading of the primary tumor is an important part of both the AJCC and Surgical Staging Systems. There is growing evidence that using the standardized uptake value (SUV) from FDG-PET can allow the differentiation of high-grade from low-grade sarcoma. For example, a retrospective study of 212 patients[16] with primary osseous and soft-tissue sarcomas showed that using an SUV cutoff of 2.5 yielded a sensitivity of 94.6% for the detection of osseous

Table 1
Relative FDG uptake in malignant and benign bone tumors[59]

		SUV	
	Relative FDG	Average	SD
Malignant	High	4.3	3.2
Osteosarcoma	High	5.2	4.2
Ewing sarcoma	Very high	9.9	5.8
Multiple myeloma	Low	1.1	0.3
Benign	Variable	2.2	1.5
Osteochondroma	Low	1.0	0.1
Enchondroma	Low	1.0	0.2
Osteoid osteoma	Low	1.5	0.1
Fibrous dysplasia	Moderate	2.1	1.0
Bone cyst	Low	1.3	0.8
Giant cell tumor	High	4.6	1.1
Chondroblastoma	Moderate	3.3	1.1
Chondromyxoid fibroma	Moderate	3.5	—

Data from Hamada K, Tomita Y, Konishi E, et al. FDG-PET evaluation of chondromyxoid fibroma of left ileum. Clin Nucl Med 2009;34:15.

sarcomas and a 94% sensitivity for the separation of high-grade from low-grade sarcomas. Similarly, another study[17] found that the degree of FDG uptake in the primary tumor (before neoadjuvant chemotherapy) provides prognostic information, as higher uptake correlated with worse outcomes.

While FDG-PET and PET/CT do perform well in the staging of sarcoma,[18] it is still unclear as to what improvement it provides over conventional imaging modalities. The latter includes radiography for initial evaluation, MR imaging for characterization of the primary tumor, CT for the detection of pulmonary metastases, and skeletal scintigraphy for the evaluation of bony metastases.[1] Two studies[19,20] found the sensitivity of FDG-PET/CT was no higher than CT alone for the detection of distant metastases, but that specificity was higher for pulmonary nodules larger than 0.5 cm and lymph nodes smaller than 1 cm. For the detection of osseous metastases, one study found that MR has a higher sensitivity than skeletal scintigraphy for the detection of bone marrow metastases but a lower sensitivity than FDG-PET.[21] Another found that FDG-PET is less sensitive than even bone scintigraphy.[22] A prospective multicenter trial involving 46 pediatric sarcoma patients,[23] however, showed that FDG-PET scanning found important additional information that had a significant impact on therapy planning compared with conventional imaging (**Fig. 1**). In particular, FDG-PET and conventional imaging were equally effective in the detection of primary tumors (accuracy 100%), but FDG-PET was superior for the detection of lymph node involvement (sensitivity 95% vs 25%, respectively) and bone manifestations (sensitivity 90% vs 57%,

respectively), whereas CT was more reliable in detecting lung metastases (sensitivity 100% vs 25%, respectively).

One of the earliest applications of FDG-PET in osseous sarcoma was for the evaluation of response to neoadjuvant chemotherapy.[24] Since then, much attention has been paid to this role, as the degree of response is a significant, independent prognostic factor for these patients.[25] At present, response is assessed during surgery through histologic evaluation. While definitive, this does not allow early response assessment and is invasive. Some early studies of FDG-PET[26] showed limited utility in this regard, but multiple studies since then have confirmed that comparison of the pretherapy FDG uptake with the posttherapy FDG uptake positively correlates with histologic outcomes.[25,27–29] Two main issues remain on this topic. The first is whether FDG-PET alone is sufficient, or whether MR imaging is also needed for proper evaluation;[30] the second is the specific method of metabolic quantitation.[31] Various studies have shown that the maximum SUV,[32] tumor to background ratio,[33] or visual analysis[34] performs the best.

Finally, FDG-PET and PET/CT have an established role in the evaluation of response to adjuvant chemotherapy and for recurrent disease.[10,18] Given the significant anatomic alterations from surgery, the metabolic information from skeletal scintigraphy and FDG-PET are invaluable. In particular, the combined anatomic and functional information in FDG-PET/CT provides for the optimal evaluation.

Figs. 2 and **3** demonstrate several examples of the utility of FDG-PET/CT in osteosarcoma.

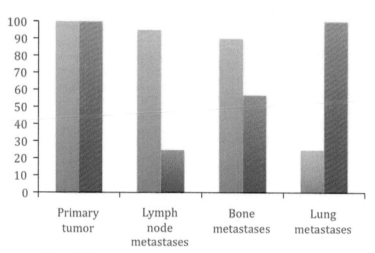

Fig. 1. Relative accuracy of FDG-PET (*blue*) versus conventional imaging (*red*) in the evaluation of osseous tumors, including osteosarcoma and Ewing sarcoma, from a large prospective trial.[23] Conventional imaging includes radiography, CT, MR imaging, and skeletal scintigraphy.

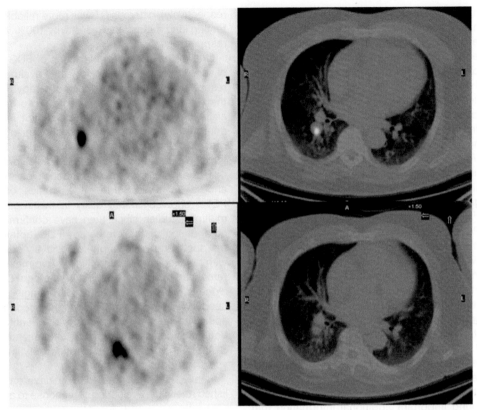

Fig. 2. A 29-year-old man with osteosarcoma. Transaxial PET (*left*) and fused PET/CT images (*right*) demonstrate intense FDG uptake in the pulmonary metastasis (*upper images*) and complete metabolic response after neoadjuvant chemotherapy (*lower images*). Note also the increased FDG uptake in the bone post therapy, which is a physiologic response.

Ewing Sarcoma

Ewing sarcoma is the second most common malignant primary bone tumor. It is thought to arise from neural crest cells and so together with the peripheral neuroectodermal tumors, makes up the Ewing sarcoma family of tumors (ESFT).[1] ESFT too is most common in childhood and adolescence. Unlike osteosarcoma, ESFT is equally found in the axial and appendicular skeleton, and when it does occur in the long bones, favors the diaphysis over the metaphysis. ESFT may also occur in the extraosseous tissues.[1]

Similar to osteosarcoma, patients with ESFT often present with ongoing (dull or aching) pain at the affected site, although swelling may be a larger component. Diagnosis ultimately requires a bone biopsy. Treatment typically involves neoadjuvant chemotherapy followed by local control. The latter may involve surgical resection, radiation therapy, or a combination of both; this is followed by additional chemotherapy.[1]

Staging follows the same systems as for osteosarcoma, and includes either the AJCC system or the Surgical Staging System (Enneking system). Again in the latter system, low-grade, localized tumors are Stage I, high-grade, localized tumors are Stage II, and metastatic tumors (regardless of grade) are Stage III.[4,13]

Imaging plays an important role in the diagnosis, staging, and posttherapy evaluation of ESFT. Radiography, MR imaging, CT, and bone scintigraphy are the conventional modalities used.[35] In general, the guidelines for the use of FDG-PET and PET/CT for ESFT are very similar to the guidelines for osteosarcoma. Indeed, this is in large part due to most studies grouping the 2 osseous sarcomas together in their analysis, which is understandable given the relatively low incidence of these tumor types. As such, FDG-PET or PET/CT has a limited role in the diagnosis of ESFT, but does have important roles in grading, staging, prognostication, evaluation of therapeutic response, and detection of recurrent disease (see **Table 1**).[14,15] Under the revised 2009 Medicare National Coverage Determinations, the initial evaluation (diagnosis and staging) is covered fully,

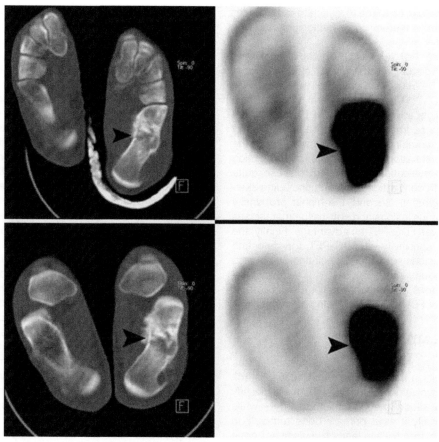

Fig. 3. A 20-year-old man with osteosarcoma of the left calcaneus. Transaxial CT (*left*) and PET (*right*) images from a pretherapy scan (*upper images*) demonstrate increased FDG uptake (SUV 5.7) in the lesion (*arrowheads*). Posttherapy PET/CT scan (*lower images*) demonstrates persistent FDG uptake (SUV 4.8), suggesting residual viable tumor. Additional evolution of bony changes are also seen on CT.

whereas subsequent evaluations (restaging and response to therapy) are covered only under the CED category.

FDG-PET and PET/CT can be used to grade the primary tumor before any intervention by evaluating the degree of FDG uptake.[16] These modalities also perform well with staging of ESFT, leading to significant treatment alterations.[23] In fact, these modalities seem to have an even more important role in ESFT than osteosarcoma because of the higher percentage of nonosseous lesions in ESFT and because the osseous lesions are better identified by FDG-PET than by skeletal scintigraphy. For instance, one study found that a staging FDG-PET scan led to 3 of 17 (18%) Ewing sarcoma patients being upstaged whereas only 1 of 38 (3%) osteosarcoma patients were upstaged.[36] This type of information is also more critical for ESFT than osteosarcoma, because it can change the treatment decision from surgery to radiation for local control. Several studies have

found that FDG-PET can detect a larger number of osseous lesions than do bone scintigraphy or gallium scans,[37,38] although whole-body MR imaging appears to do so as well.[39] The main downfall of FDG-PET or PET/CT for staging of ESFT is in evaluation of pulmonary metastases. Again, several studies show that FDG-PET does not perform as well as high-resolution CT for this purpose, especially for nodules smaller than 1 cm.[19,20,37,40]

As for osteosarcoma, several studies have shown that FDG-PET and PET/CT can be used to accurately monitor response to neoadjuvant chemotherapy. This imaging provides a noninvasive way to monitor therapeutic response at an early time point and correlates positively with histologic evaluation at surgery.[31,41,42] Again, this is potentially more important for ESFT than for osteosarcoma, given that not all patients undergo surgical resection for local control. If patients do not respond well to neoadjuvant chemotherapy the decision can be made to switch to radiation for local control, thereby preventing unnecessary surgery.

Response to additional therapy, including surgery, radiation, and adjuvant chemotherapy, can also be reliably performed with FDG-PET and PET/CT.[15] Moreover, several studies have shown a slight advantage to FDG-PET in detection of recurrences from ESFT.[43,44] The latter is likely due to a combination of 3 factors. First, the anatomic alteration from surgery and radiation can make evaluation of recurrent disease quite difficult with conventional imaging (including skeletal scintigraphy). Second, the higher propensity of nonosseous lesions and soft-tissue metastases in ESFT gives FDG-PET an advantage. Finally, the increased sensitivity of FDG-PET for detecting osseous lesions over skeletal scintigraphy is also advantageous.

Figs. 4 to **6** demonstrate several examples of the utility of FDG-PET/CT in Ewing sarcoma.

MULTIPLE MYELOMA

Multiple myeloma (MM) is a malignancy of the plasma cells in the bone marrow. Because of the marrow involvement, some authorities classify MM as a blood (hematologic) disorder, while others classify it as a primary bone tumor.[45] In either case, the disease leads to significant bone involvement in the vast majority (>90%) of patients.[3] According to the 2009 American Cancer Society estimates, approximately 20,580 new cases were expected in 2009. The estimated number of deaths in 2009 from this malignancy is 10,580.[5]

The peak incidence of MM is in the older population, 50 to 70 years old. MM rarely occurs in people younger than 30 years. Patients may be asymptomatic, but usually present with pain at the primary site of involvement. This pain is due to unchecked lytic activity surrounding the pathologic plasma cells, likely from release of local factors stimulating osteoclasts. These lytic lesions are the hallmark of MM and may appear in any bone, but most commonly affect the spine, pelvis, and skull.[45]

Other associated entities include solitary plasmacytomas and monoclonal gammopathy of undetermined significance (MGUS). The former occurs when the abnormal plasma cells form only a solitary lesion, and the latter occurs when no lesion is present at all. Both these entities may subsequently go on to develop MM.[45] Traditional treatment options include chemotherapy and radiation therapy, with surgery having essentially no role. However, many new therapies are being evaluated including autologous bone marrow transplantation, gene therapy, immunotherapy, and several new therapeutic drug

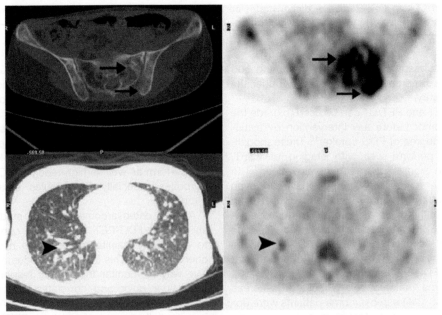

Fig. 4. A 21-year-old woman with Ewing sarcoma. Transaxial CT (*left*) and PET images (*right*) demonstrate the primary pelvic tumor (*arrows*) as well as pulmonary metastases (*arrowheads*). The bony involvement is intensely FDG avid, as is typical for Ewing sarcoma, whereas the pulmonary nodules are less FDG avid given their smaller size and resultant volume-averaging effects.

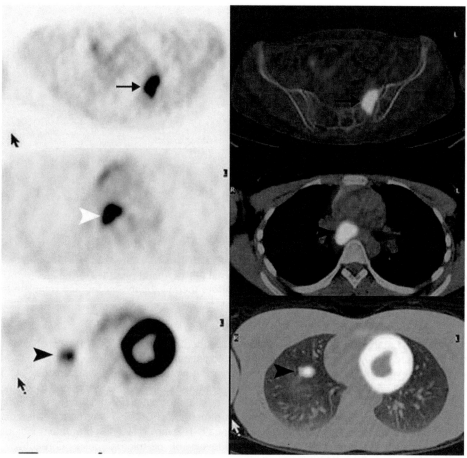

Fig. 5. A 24-year-old woman with Ewing sarcoma. Transaxial PET (*left*) and fused PET/CT images (*right*) show the primary pelvic tumor (*black arrows*), as well as mediastinal lymph node (*white arrow*) and pulmonary metastases (*black arrowheads*), all with intense FDG uptake.

combinations.[45] Other therapeutic regimens include bisphosphonate therapy, kyphoplasty, vertebroplasty, and novel agents to suppress osteoclastic bone resorption.[3]

Staging of MM involves laboratory studies to determine the hemoglobin value, serum calcium, and monoclonal protein levels, and imaging to determine the extent of lytic bone lesions. As such, imaging plays an important role in this malignancy. Various modalities have been used or studied in MM including radiography, CT, MR imaging, and FDG-PET and PET/CT. The International Myeloma Working Group consensus statement and guidelines regarding the current role of imaging techniques in the diagnosis and monitoring of MM[46] states that conventional radiography still remains the "gold standard" of the staging procedure of newly diagnosed and relapsed myeloma patients. A skeletal survey using a series of plain films covering the chest, pelvis, bilateral humeri and femora, skull, and

vertebral column traditionally formed the mainstay of myeloma imaging.[45,47] However, early-stage disease and overlapping structures are limitations to plain films that cross-sectional imaging can overcome. MR imaging gives information complementary to skeletal survey, and is recommended in MM patients with normal conventional radiography and in all patients with an apparently solitary plasmacytoma of bone. In particular, whole-body MR imaging has been shown to be even more sensitive than CT, as marrow infiltrates are displayed before osseous destructions occur.[47] Bone scintigraphy and dual-energy X-ray absorptiometry scans are not recommended. Given the nature of this malignancy, multimodality PET/CT seems to be a logical choice for evaluation of this process. Indeed, there is growing evidence to support the use of FDG-PET and PET/CT for the diagnosis/staging, prognosis, assessment of complications, and response evaluation in patients with MM.[48–50]

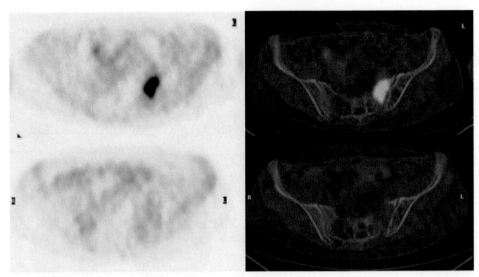

Fig. 6. A 24-year-old woman with Ewing sarcoma. Transaxial PET (*left*) and fused PET/CT images (*right*) demonstrate intense FDG uptake in the primary pelvic tumor before therapy (*upper images*) and complete metabolic response after neoadjuvant chemotherapy (*lower images*).

For diagnosis and staging, the optimal imaging modality would accurately identify all areas of bony involvement without resulting in too high a false-positive rate. As mentioned earlier, the traditional skeletal survey has a tendency to understage the patient as early-stage disease and certain anatomic regions are not well analyzed. Several studies have now shown that CT, MR imaging, and FDG-PET/CT result in improved staging (increased sensitivity) of patients with MM.[49,51,52] The primary advantage of CT is its speed. Intramedullary lesions are clearly seen as long as they are located in long bones where they are surrounded by fat. Diffuse bone marrow infiltration and intravertebral lesions, however, are difficult to detect with whole-body CT in the absence of frank destruction of cancellous bone. MR imaging is most sensitive to both diffuse bone marrow involvement and solid plasma cell tumors.

Head-to-head comparison of FDG-PET and whole-body MR imaging found that MR imaging performed better than PET in the assessment of disease activity, having a higher sensitivity and specificity. The positive predictive value of whole-body MR imaging in the assessment of active disease was high, at 88%. When used in combination and with concordant findings, PET and whole-body MR imaging were found to have a specificity and positive predictive value of 100%, which may be of value to clinicians assessing the effectiveness of aggressive and expensive treatment regimens.[53] Also, because whole-body MR imaging is not a typically performed

procedure, FDG-PET/CT is more available and logistically easier.[54] By contrast, FDG-PET/CT alone would miss small lytic lesions.[55]

Moreover, FDG-PET appears to deliver prognostic information.[56] In a survey of 239 untreated patients,[57] FDG-PET correlated with prognostically relevant baseline parameters including high levels of $\beta2$-microglobulin, C-reactive protein, and lactate dehydrogenase. The presence of more than 3 FDG-avid focal lesions was related to fundamental features of myeloma biology and genomics, and was the leading independent parameter associated with inferior overall and event-free survival. Similarly, complete FDG suppression in focal lesions before transplantation conferred significantly better outcomes and was only opposed by gene expression profiling-defined high-risk status. These results suggest that myeloma survival can be improved by altering treatment in patients in whom FDG suppression cannot be achieved after induction therapy. FDG-PET is also useful for evaluation of nonsecretory myeloma. Residual or recurrent disease after therapy, especially extramedullary disease, is a poor prognostic factor.

FDG-PET/CT appears to outperform whole-body MR imaging in assessing response to therapy.[49,51] An important caveat to this is that the original tumor (pretherapy) requires high FDG uptake. In such cases response assessment is effective with FDG-PET and PET/CT, as the FDG uptake will decrease after successful chemotherapy or stem cell transplant;[47,50] this has also been shown in plasmacytomas.[58] Of note, the rate of resolution of FDG uptake post treatment does not necessarily imply an adverse prognosis.

Fig. 7 demonstrates the utility of FDG-PET/CT for MM.

BENIGN TUMORS OF BONE

Benign primary tumors of bone are a heterogeneous group of disorders including (in rough order of prevalence) osteochondroma, enchondroma, osteoid osteoma, fibrous dysplasia, aneurysmal bone cyst, giant cell tumors, chondroblastoma, and chondromyxoid fibroma. Some, such as giant cell tumors and fibrous dysplasia, may transform into malignancy. Others are strictly benign, but nonetheless can lead to significant local effects such as pain and pathologic fractures.

The imaging evaluation of benign bone tumors is primarily restricted to anatomic imaging, including radiography, CT, and MR imaging. However, functional imaging with MDP bone scintigraphy is not infrequently used to help differentiate benign from malignant processes when conventional imaging findings are equivocal. Bone scintigraphy is also used to conveniently survey the whole skeleton, for instance to differentiate monostotic from polyostotic fibrous dysplasia.

FDG-PET and PET/CT are not typically used to evaluate benign primary tumors of bone, primarily because of the proven utility of conventional imaging and the lower specificity but higher cost for FDG-PET.[59] As such, the utility of FDG-PET in evaluating these lesions is less important prospectively, but important retrospectively, as various benign lesions are often incidentally seen on CT. **Table 1** summarizes the relative and absolute degree of FDG uptake in various benign bone tumors. Unfortunately only a few studies have been published on this topic, and the results are somewhat inconclusive. For instance, several studies have shown that one can use FDG-PET to differentiate benign from malignant osseous lesions.[59–62] In particular, SUV assessment of FDG accumulation within osseous lesions was superior to subjective visual analysis for discriminating benign from malignant lesions.[62] Using an SUV cutoff value of 2, 14 of 15 malignant lesions were categorized correctly versus 12 of 15

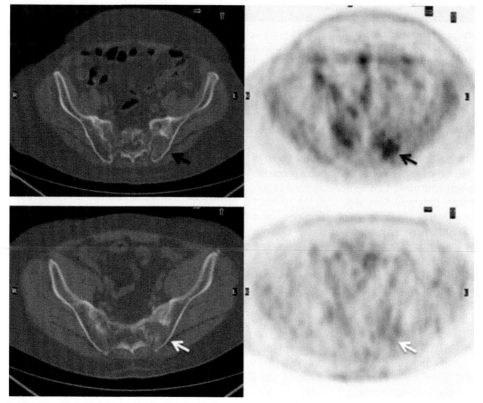

Fig. 7. A 66-year-old man with multiple myeloma. Pretherapy scan (*upper images*) shows a lytic lesion in the left sacrum with increased FDG uptake (*black arrows*). The postradiation therapy scan (*lower images*) shows resolution of FDG uptake, but a persistent lytic lesion on CT (*white arrows*).

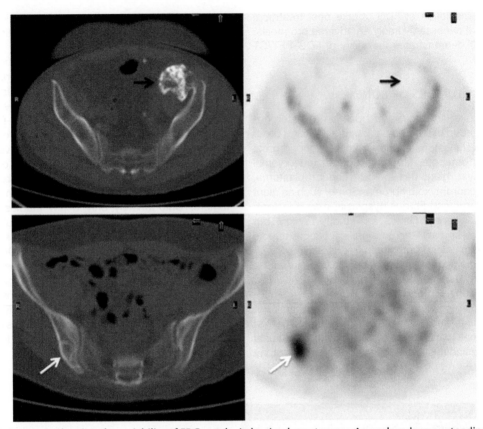

Fig. 8. Image set showing the variability of FDG uptake in benign bone tumors. An enchondroma extending from the left anterior iliac bone shows no increased FDG uptake (*upper images, black arrows*). Fibrous dysplasia in the right posterior iliac bone shows intense FDG uptake (*lower images, white arrows*).

correctly categorized by means of subjective image evaluation; 4 of 5 benign lesions were categorized correctly with both techniques.

By contrast, other studies showed that there is a high degree of variability in FDG uptake across both benign and malignant tumors of bone, such that reliable differentiation was difficult without correlation with other imaging findings and history.[63] For instance, enchondromas do not generally show significant FDG uptake, but an actively proliferating enchondroma was found to have intense FDG uptake.[64] Similarly, fibrous dysplasia and giant cell tumors can have prominent FDG uptake.[59] However, based on one study, the use of CT significantly improved differentiation over PET alone.[65] The same study showed that although PET/CT more commonly differentiated benign from malignant primary bone lesions compared with conventional radiographs, this difference was not significant.

Fig. 8 shows 2 examples of enchondroma and fibrous dysplasia, demonstrating the variability in FDG uptake within benign bone lesions.

SUMMARY

Primary bone tumors are a heterogeneous group of diseases including malignant and benign variants. The former includes osteosarcoma and the ESFT, while the latter includes several entities such as osteochondroma, enchondroma, aneurysmal bone cyst, and fibrous dysplasia. MM is a hematologic malignancy that primarily presents in bone.

Imaging is critical for the proper staging, management, and posttherapy evaluation of these patients. While conventional imaging such as radiography, CT, MR imaging, and bone scintigraphy remain the mainstay, there is growing evidence for the use of FDG-PET and PET/CT in the grading, staging, prognostication, evaluation of therapeutic response, and detection of recurrent disease. Conventional imaging appears to perform well for initial diagnosis and staging, but subsequent evaluation is hampered by anatomic alterations from surgery and radiation. By contrast, FDG-PET and PET/CT have a more limited role for staging, but outperform conventional imaging for restaging, response to therapy, and evaluation of recurrent disease. In particular, the metabolic information from PET is critical for the evaluation of response to neoadjuvant chemotherapy in sarcoma and for response assessment in myeloma.

Benign tumors of bone may have considerable overlap of FDG uptake with malignant disorders, but carefully combining the anatomic and metabolic information together with the history should allow proper differentiation of malignant from benign tumors. The role of FDG-PET and PET/CT will continue to expand and transform as the number of long-term studies on their efficacy are published.

REFERENCES

1. Heare T, Hensley MA, Dell'Orfano S. Bone tumors: osteosarcoma and Ewing's sarcoma. Curr Opin Pediatr 2009;21:365.
2. Simon MA, Finn HA. Diagnostic strategy for bone and soft-tissue tumors. Instr Course Lect 1994;43:527.
3. Roodman GD. Skeletal imaging and management of bone disease. Hematology Am Soc Hematol Educ Program 2008;1:313.
4. Pommersheim WJ, Chew FS. Imaging, diagnosis, and staging of bone tumors: a primer. Semin Roentgenol 2004;39:361.
5. Jemal A, Siegel R, Ward E, et al. Cancer statistics, 2009. CA Cancer J Clin 2009;59:225.
6. Seeger LL, Gold RH, Chandnani VP. Diagnostic imaging of osteosarcoma. Clin Orthop Relat Res 1991;254.
7. Focacci C, Lattanzi R, Iadeluca ML, et al. Nuclear medicine in primary bone tumors. Eur J Radiol 1998;27(Suppl 1):S123.
8. Abdel-Dayem HM. The role of nuclear medicine in primary bone and soft tissue tumors. Semin Nucl Med 1997;27:355.
9. Gambhir SS. Molecular imaging of cancer with positron emission tomography. Nat Rev Cancer 2002;2:683.
10. Kumar R, Chauhan A, Vellimana AK, et al. Role of PET/PET-CT in the management of sarcomas. Expert Rev Anticancer Ther 2006;6:1241.
11. Beyer T, Townsend DW, Blodgett TM. Dual-modality PET/CT tomography for clinical oncology. Q J Nucl Med 2002;46:24.
12. Gerth HU, Juergens KU, Dirksen U, et al. Significant benefit of multimodal imaging: PET/CT compared with PET alone in staging and follow-up of patients with Ewing tumors. J Nucl Med 1932;48:2007.
13. Heck RK Jr, Stacy GS, Flaherty MJ, et al. A comparison study of staging systems for bone sarcomas. Clin Orthop Relat Res 2003;415:64.

14. Meyer JS, Nadel HR, Marina N, et al. Imaging guidelines for children with Ewing sarcoma and osteosarcoma: a report from the Children's Oncology Group Bone Tumor Committee. Pediatr Blood Cancer 2008;51:163.
15. McCarville MB, Christie R, Daw NC, et al. PET/CT in the evaluation of childhood sarcomas. AJR Am J Roentgenol 2005;184:1293.
16. Charest M, Hickeson M, Lisbona R, et al. FDG PET/CT imaging in primary osseous and soft tissue sarcomas: a retrospective review of 212 cases. Eur J Nucl Med Mol Imaging 2009. [Epub ahead of print].
17. Franzius C, Bielack S, Flege S, et al. Prognostic significance of (18)F-FDG and (99m)Tc-methylene diphosphonate uptake in primary osteosarcoma. J Nucl Med 2002;43:1012.
18. Benz MR, Tchekmedyian N, Eilber FC, et al. Utilization of positron emission tomography in the management of patients with sarcoma. Curr Opin Oncol 2009;21:345.
19. Kleis M, Daldrup-Link H, Matthay K, et al. Diagnostic value of PET/CT for the staging and restaging of pediatric tumors. Eur J Nucl Med Mol Imaging 2009;36:23.
20. Franzius C, Daldrup-Link HE, Sciuk J, et al. FDG-PET for detection of pulmonary metastases from malignant primary bone tumors: comparison with spiral CT. Ann Oncol 2001;12:479.
21. Daldrup-Link HE, Franzius C, Link TM, et al. Whole-body MR imaging for detection of bone metastases in children and young adults: comparison with skeletal scintigraphy and FDG PET. AJR Am J Roentgenol 2001;177:229.
22. Franzius C, Sciuk J, Daldrup-Link HE, et al. FDG-PET for detection of osseous metastases from malignant primary bone tumours: comparison with bone scintigraphy. Eur J Nucl Med 2000;27:1305.
23. Volker T, Denecke T, Steffen I, et al. Positron emission tomography for staging of pediatric sarcoma patients: results of a prospective multicenter trial. J Clin Oncol 2007;25:5435.
24. Schulte M, Brecht-Krauss D, Werner M, et al. Evaluation of neoadjuvant therapy response of osteogenic sarcoma using FDG-PET. J Nucl Med 1999;40:1637.
25. Hawkins DS, Conrad EU 3rd, Butrynski JE, et al. [F-18]-fluorodeoxy-D-glucose-positron emission tomography response is associated with outcome for extremity osteosarcoma in children and young adults. Cancer 2009;115:3519.
26. Huang TL, Liu RS, Chen TH, et al. Comparison between F-18-FDG positron emission tomography and histology for the assessment of tumor necrosis rates in primary osteosarcoma. J Chin Med Assoc 2006;69:372.
27. Hamada K, Tomita Y, Inoue A, et al. Evaluation of chemotherapy response in osteosarcoma with FDG-PET. Ann Nucl Med 2009;23:89.

28. Dutour A, Decouvelaere AV, Monteil J, et al. ^{18}F-FDG PET SUV$_{max}$ correlates with osteosarcoma histologic response to neoadjuvant chemotherapy: preclinical evaluation in an orthotopic rat model. J Nucl Med 2009;50:1533.

29. Costelloe CM, Macapinlac HA, Madewell JE, et al. ^{18}F-FDG PET/CT as an indicator of progression-free and overall survival in osteosarcoma. J Nucl Med 2009;50:340.

30. Cheon GJ, Kim MS, Lee JA, et al. Prediction model of chemotherapy response in osteosarcoma by ^{18}F-FDG PET and MRI. J Nucl Med 2009;50:1435.

31. Schuetze SM. Utility of positron emission tomography in sarcomas. Curr Opin Oncol 2006; 18:369.

32. Benz MR, Evilevitch V, Allen-Auerbach MS, et al. Treatment monitoring by ^{18}F-FDG PET/CT in patients with sarcomas: interobserver variability of quantitative parameters in treatment-induced changes in histopathologically responding and nonresponding tumors. J Nucl Med 2008;49:1038.

33. Ye Z, Zhu J, Tian M, et al. Response of osteogenic sarcoma to neoadjuvant therapy: evaluated by ^{18}F-FDG-PET. Ann Nucl Med 2008;22:475.

34. Nair N, Ali A, Green AA, et al. Response of osteosarcoma to chemotherapy. Evaluation with F-18 FDG-PET Scans. Clin Positron Imaging 2000;3:79.

35. Mar WA, Taljanovic MS, Bagatell R, et al. Update on imaging and treatment of Ewing sarcoma family tumors: what the radiologist needs to know. J Comput Assist Tomogr 2008;32:108.

36. Kneisl JS, Patt JC, Johnson JC, et al. Is PET useful in detecting occult nonpulmonary metastases in pediatric bone sarcomas? Clin Orthop Relat Res 2006; 450:101.

37. Gyorke T, Zajic T, Lange A, et al. Impact of FDG PET for staging of Ewing sarcomas and primitive neuroectodermal tumours. Nucl Med Commun 2006;27:17.

38. Hung GU, Tan TS, Kao CH, et al. Multiple skeletal metastases of Ewing's sarcoma demonstrated on FDG-PET and compared with bone and gallium scans. Kaohsiung J Med Sci 2000;16:315.

39. Furth C, Amthauer H, Denecke T, et al. Impact of whole-body MRI and FDG-PET on staging and assessment of therapy response in a patient with Ewing sarcoma. Pediatr Blood Cancer 2006;47:607.

40. Iagaru A, Chawla S, Menendez L, et al. ^{18}F-FDG PET and PET/CT for detection of pulmonary metastases from musculoskeletal sarcomas. Nucl Med Commun 2006;27:795.

41. Hawkins DS, Schuetze SM, Butrynski JE, et al. [^{18}F]Fluorodeoxyglucose positron emission tomography predicts outcome for Ewing sarcoma family of tumors. J Clin Oncol 2005;23:8828.

42. Franzius C, Sciuk J, Brinkschmidt C, et al. Evaluation of chemotherapy response in primary bone tumors with F-18 FDG positron emission tomography compared with histologically assessed tumor necrosis. Clin Nucl Med 2000;25:874.

43. Franzius C, Schulte M, Hillmann A, et al. [Clinical value of positron emission tomography (PET) in the diagnosis of bone and soft tissue tumors. 3rd Interdisciplinary Consensus Conference "PET in Oncology": results of the Bone and Soft Tissue Study Group]. Chirurg 2001;72:1071 [in German].

44. Franzius C, Daldrup-Link HE, Wagner-Bohn A, et al. FDG-PET for detection of recurrences from malignant primary bone tumors: comparison with conventional imaging. Ann Oncol 2002;13:157.

45. White TB, Caldwell D, Hall-Rollins J. Multiple myeloma. Radiol Technol 2005;76:379.

46. Dimopoulos M, Terpos E, Comenzo RL, et al. International myeloma working group consensus statement and guidelines regarding the current role of imaging techniques in the diagnosis and monitoring of multiple myeloma. Leukemia 2009; 23:1545.

47. Baur-Melnyk A, Reiser MF. Multiple myeloma. Semin Musculoskelet Radiol 2009;13:111.

48. Winterbottom AP, Shaw AS. Imaging patients with myeloma. Clin Radiol 2009;64:1.

49. Delorme S, Baur-Melnyk A. Imaging in multiple myeloma. Eur J Radiol 2009;70:401.

50. Bredella MA, Steinbach L, Caputo G, et al. Value of FDG PET in the assessment of patients with multiple myeloma. AJR Am J Roentgenol 2005; 184:1199.

51. Lutje S, de Rooy JW, Croockewit S, et al. Role of radiography, MRI and FDG-PET/CT in diagnosing, staging and therapeutical evaluation of patients with multiple myeloma. Ann Hematol 2009;88:1161.

52. Schirrmeister H, Bommer M, Buck AK, et al. Initial results in the assessment of multiple myeloma using ^{18}F-FDG PET. Eur J Nucl Med Mol Imaging 2002;29:361.

53. Shortt CP, Gleeson TG, Breen KA, et al. Whole-Body MRI versus PET in assessment of multiple myeloma disease activity. AJR Am J Roentgenol 2009;192:980.

54. Zamagni E, Nanni C, Patriarca F, et al. A prospective comparison of ^{18}F-fluorodeoxyglucose positron emission tomography-computed tomography, magnetic resonance imaging and whole-body planar radiographs in the assessment of bone disease in newly diagnosed multiple myeloma. Haematologica 2007;92:50.

55. Breyer RJ 3rd, Mulligan ME, Smith SE, et al. Comparison of imaging with FDG PET/CT with other imaging modalities in myeloma. Skeletal Radiol 2006;35:632.

56. Bartel TB, Haessler J, Brown TL, et al. F18-fluoro-deoxyglucose positron emission tomography in the context of other imaging techniques and prognostic factors in multiple myeloma. Blood 2009; 114:2068.

57. Durie BG, Waxman AD, D'Agnolo A, et al. Whole-body (18)F-FDG PET identifies high-risk myeloma. J Nucl Med 2002;43:1457.

58. Kim PJ, Hicks RJ, Wirth A, et al. Impact of ^{18}F-fluorodeoxyglucose positron emission tomography before and after definitive radiation therapy in patients with apparently solitary plasmacytoma. Int J Radiat Oncol Biol Phys 2009;74:740.

59. Aoki J, Watanabe H, Shinozaki T, et al. FDG PET of primary benign and malignant bone tumors: standardized uptake value in 52 lesions. Radiology 2001;219:774.

60. Aoki J, Inoue T, Tomiyoshi K, et al. Nuclear imaging of bone tumors: FDG-PET. Semin Musculoskelet Radiol 2001;5:183.

61. Aoki J, Watanabe H, Shinozaki T, et al. FDG-PET for preoperative differential diagnosis between benign and malignant soft tissue masses. Skeletal Radiol 2003;32:133.

62. Dehdashti F, Siegel BA, Griffeth LK, et al. Benign versus malignant intraosseous lesions: discrimination by means of PET with 2-[F-18]fluoro-2-deoxy-D-glucose. Radiology 1996;200:243.

63. Maeda T, Tateishi U, Terauchi T, et al. Unsuspected bone and soft tissue lesions identified at cancer screening using positron emission tomography. Jpn J Clin Oncol 2007;37:207.

64. Dobert N, Menzel C, Ludwig R, et al. Enchondroma: a benign osseous lesion with high F-18 FDG uptake. Clin Nucl Med 2002;27:695.

65. Strobel K, Exner UE, Stumpe KD, et al. The additional value of CT images interpretation in the differential diagnosis of benign vs. malignant primary bone lesions with ^{18}F-FDG-PET/CT. Eur J Nucl Med Mol Imaging 2008;35:2000.

FDG-PET and PET/CT for Evaluating Soft Tissue Sarcomas

Cristina Nanni, MD*, Stefano Fanti, MD

KEYWORDS

- Positron emission tomography • FDG
- Soft tissue sarcomas

GENERAL OVERVIEW ON SARCOMAS

The group of sarcoma tumors is heterogeneous and includes 2 main groups of neoplasms: soft tissue sarcomas and bone sarcomas.

Soft tissue sarcomas have mesodermal origin and usually begin in the muscle, fat, fibrous tissue, blood vessels, or other supporting tissue of the body. These sarcomas constitute approximately 1% of adult malignancies and 7% of pediatric malignancies. The most frequent types are fibrosarcoma and malignant fibrous histiocytoma among those originating from fibrous tissue; liposarcoma originating from fatty tissue; leiomyosarcoma from smooth muscle; rhabdomyosarcoma from skeletal muscle; angiosarcoma, lymphangiosarcoma, and Kaposi sarcoma from blood and lymph vessels; hemangiopericytoma from perivascular tissue; synovial sarcoma from synovial tissue; schwannoma from peripheral nerves; and gastrointestinal stromal tumor (GIST) from mesenchymal cells.

Bone sarcomas are even rarer, representing only 0.2% of all new cancer diagnoses, with a biphasic pattern including a peak in adolescence (primary sarcomas) and a peak in the elderly (secondary sarcomas associated with Paget disease and irradiated bones).

Bone sarcomas basically include the group of Ewing sarcoma and osteosarcoma. The group of Ewing sarcomas includes Ewing tumors of bone or Ewing sarcoma of bone, extraosseous Ewing tumors, primitive neuroectodermal tumors (PNETs) or peripheral neuroepithelioma, and Askin tumors (PNETs of the chest wall). These tumors come from the same type of stem cell.

Most soft tissue sarcomas are sporadic, with no specific causal agent. In some cases, however, a predisposing factor can be recognized, such as exposure to alkylating chemotherapeutic agents, Paget disease, areas of bone infarction, irradiated bones, neurofibromatosis, tuberous sclerosis, Gardner syndrome, and Li-Fraumeni syndrome.

Soft tissue sarcomas arise predominantly in the abdomen and in the extremities, whereas bone sarcomas may arise in any bone and within any region of a given bone. However, osteosarcoma arises most frequently in the long bones of the lower extremities, whereas Ewing sarcoma has a predilection for the long tubular bones, the flat bones of the pelvis, and the ribs.

Usually the clinical presentation of patients with soft tissue sarcomas depends on the primary tumor site, whereas most patients with bone sarcoma present with localized pain. The diagnosis of sarcoma arises after a computed tomography (CT) scan for soft tissue sarcomas, a magnetic resonance (MR) imaging scan for bone sarcomas, and a targeted biopsy. The disease staging is performed with satisfactory accuracy, mainly with CT, especially for the evaluation of lung metastasis.

The prognosis of these neoplasms is strongly related to several factors, the important ones being the extent of the disease at diagnosis, the grade of the tumor, the age of the patient, the presence of microscopically positive margins after resection,

Department of Nuclear Medicine, Azienda Ospedaliero-Universitaria di Bologna Policlinico S.Orsola-Malpighi, Via Massarenti n. 9, 40138 Bologna, Italy
* Corresponding author.
E-mail address: cristina.nanni@aosp.bo.it

PET Clin 5 (2010) 341–347
doi:10.1016/j.cpet.2010.04.005

the presence of metastasis at disease diagnosis, and a long duration of symptoms before the diagnosis.

The treatment of sarcomas relies basically on surgery, which is aimed at completely eradicating the disease. However, it is possible to increase patient survival by combining surgery with chemotherapy and radiation therapy (adjuvant or neoadjuvant), to facilitate surgical excision of large tumors, or to consolidate local treatment after surgical resection.

Follow-up for patients successfully treated for soft tissue sarcomas or bone sarcomas requires an understanding of the relationship between the risk of recurrence and the amount of time elapsed after treatment. Long-term follow-up studies demonstrate that approximately 80% of patients who develop recurrent disease do so within the first 3 years after therapy and that patients who are alive without recurrence at 5 and 10 years after therapy apparently still carry a risk for a subsequent late recurrence.[1]

All surveillance strategies include physical examination, appropriate imaging of the primary site of the tumor, and chest imaging for the risk of lung metastasis.

Since the greater share of sarcomas are intermediate- or high-grade tumors, positron emission tomography (PET) can be used as an additional and valuable imaging method to integrate the standard diagnostic techniques (mainly CT and MR).

There are multiple indications to perform a PET scan in patients affected by sarcomas. Several articles were published recently, and from this number, PET can be successfully used for predicting the prognosis, for staging the disease, and for assessing the response to therapy.[2] [18]F fluorodeoxyglucose (FDG) seems to be the most accurate radiopharmaceutical. However, many other tracers have been tested with positive results, among which the most important are ^{11}C choline, ^{18}F fluorothymidine (FLT), and ^{11}C methionine.

FDG-PET: A PROGNOSTIC TEST?

Because of the general poor prognosis, it is important to find out as many prognostic factors as possible when evaluating a patient affected by sarcoma, to choose the best therapeutic approach, and to correctly schedule the follow-up examinations.

Many investigators analyzed the possible role of FDG-PET/CT in predicting the prognosis when it is performed at diagnosis and after the presurgical chemotherapy.

Eary and colleagues,[3] for example, evaluated a series of 238 patients affected by different kinds of sarcomas who underwent FDG-PET/CT before therapy (chemotherapy or surgical resection) and compared the PET result with the overall survival and the disease-free survival. PET images were analyzed in terms of standardized uptake value (SUV_{max}) and spatial heterogeneity of FDG distribution within the primary mass, because it was noticed that biologic heterogeneity (including proliferation, necrosis, noncellular accumulations such as matrix material and fibrous tissue, differences in blood flow, cellular metabolism, oxygenation, and receptorial expression) is a very important feature of malignant tumors. The investigators found that SUV_{max} (an index of malignancy) and FDG heterogeneous distribution can distinguish between higher risk patients and lower risk patients and that it is therefore possible to recognize 2 groups of patients with different prognoses on the basis of FDG-PET/CT results.

Similar results were obtained by Lisle and colleagues,[4] who considered the SUV_{max} in FDG-PET before therapy in a series of 44 patients affected by synovial sarcoma. These investigators found that pretherapy SUV_{max} was predictive for overall survival and progression-free survival (PFS). Furthermore, patients with SUV_{max} greater than 4.35 at diagnosis had a decreased disease-free survival and were therefore at risk for focal recurrences and metastatic disease.

The role of FDG-PET/CT in the evaluation of leiomyosarcomas of the uterus was not widely analyzed in literature, probably because of the rare incidence of this type of malignancy. However, Punt and colleagues[5] studied the predictive value of SUV_{max} in a series of patients with leiomyosarcoma at diagnosis, revealing that apparently in leiomyosarcoma, the SUV_{max} from FDG-PET/CT is a likely predictor of tumor behavior. The results of this study suggest that a large (by greatest dimension) intermediate-grade tumor is expected to have the same predicted outcome as a high-grade tumor and should be treated in the same manner, because they share the same prognosis by definition of tumor grade. Improvements made in the clinical treatment of leiomyosarcomas by use of FDG-PET/CT imaging data may lead to an increase in patient survival.

PET AND RESPONSE TO THERAPY

In case a neoadjuvant chemotherapy is indicated, the noninvasive evaluation of the response to therapy is difficult with standard methods because the mass size usually does not change much even in responder patients.

Evilevitch and colleagues[6] found that the decrease of SUV after neoadjuvant chemotherapy is strongly correlated to the pathologic response to therapy. These investigators evaluated a series of 42 patients with resectable biopsy-proven soft tissue sarcomas who underwent a FDG-PET/CT before and after therapy and found that in histopathological responders, the reduction of FDG uptake was significantly greater than in nonresponders. Using a 60% decrease in tumor FDG uptake as a threshold, the sensitivity was 100% and the specificity was 71% for assessment of histopathological response.

Shinto and colleagues[7] proved that FDG-PET/CT may predict the response to imatinib as early as 24 hours after the administration of the first dose of the drug in a patient affected by GIST, with a significant decrease in SUV_{max} from 13.45 to 4.26.

Prior and colleagues[8] used the FDG-PET/CT imaging to predict the response to sunitinib in patients affected by GIST. Tumor metabolism was assessed with FDG-PET/CT before and after the first 4 weeks of sunitinib therapy in 23 patients who received 1 to 12 cycles of sunitinib therapy.

PFS turned out to correlate with early FDG-PET/CT metabolic response; early FDG-PET/CT response was stratified in metabolic partial response, metabolically stable disease, or metabolically progressive disease, with a median PFS rate of 29, 16, and 4 weeks, respectively. Similarly, when a single FDG-PET/CT positive/negative result was considered after 4 weeks of sunitinib, the median PFS was 29 weeks for SUVs less than 8 g/mL versus 4 weeks for SUVs of 8 g/mL or greater (P<.0001). None of the patients with metabolically progressive disease subsequently responded according to Response Evaluation Criteria In Solid Tumors criteria. The investigators concluded that FDG-PET/CT is useful for early assessment of treatment response and for the prediction of clinical outcome. Thus, it offers opportunities to individualize and optimize patient therapy (**Figs. 1** and **2**).

These results are concordant with many studies in literature. However, the semiquantitative method chosen is important. The interobserver

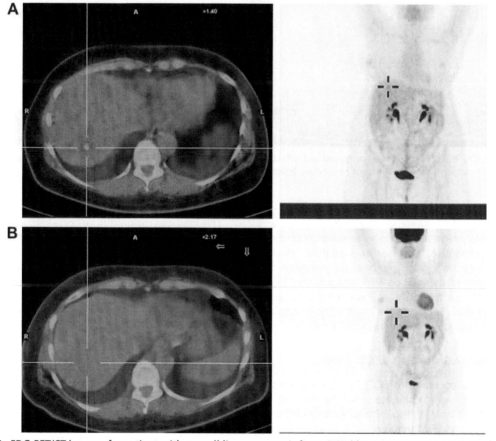

Fig. 1. FDG-PET/CT image of a patient with a small liver metastasis from GIST (the primary mass was excised). (*A*) Small liver positive lesion. (*B*) Lack of evidence of metabolically active disease in the FDG-PET/CT image 1 month after the beginning of imatinib administration is consistent with complete response to therapy.

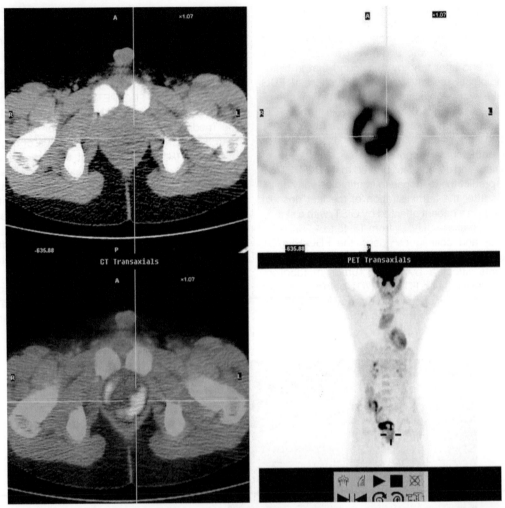

Fig. 2. FDG-PET/CT image of a young patient affected by intraprostatic rhabdomyosarcoma. The scan shows a big primary mass with no evidence of secondary lesions.

variability of the semiquantitative methods seems to be very high according to a research by Benz and colleagues.[9] These investigators studied which method was the best to measure the response to therapy on PET images and found that SUV_{max} and SUV_{peak}, not tumour-to-background ratio, provided the most robust measurements of glucose metabolism in sarcomas.

PET IN STAGING AND RESTAGING

The good accuracy of FDG-PET/CT for staging and restaging malignancies led to the idea of testing this imaging modality for patients affected by sarcomas. Furthermore, PET is a single-step examination allowing the evaluation of the whole body, and it is not difficult to include even the extremities in the field of view if needed.

This idea was mainly due for bone sarcomas, and therefore, most of the patient populations taken into consideration in published literature are children. All the studies are designed comparing the result of an FDG-PET/CT scan to conventional imaging modalities (MR, CT, bone scintigraphy, ultrasound [US], and chest radiography) to assess the accuracy of PET in determining the extension of disease at staging and restaging.

Völker and colleagues[10] evaluated 46 pediatric patients affected by Ewing sarcoma, osteosarcoma, or rhabdomyosarcoma in a multicenter study. All the patients underwent an FDG-PET/CT procedure for staging the disease, and its result was compared with those of standard imaging procedures. FDG-PET/CT and conventional imaging were equally accurate for detecting the primary tumor (100% accuracy). PET was superior in assessing lymph node involvement and bone manifestations, whereas CT turned out to be more accurate for the detection of pulmonary metastasis (see **Fig. 2; Fig. 3**). Therefore, FDG-PET/CT has a very significant effect on the management of pediatric sarcomas compared with conventional imaging.

Similar results were obtained by Tateishi and colleagues[11] on a patient population of 117 patients. These investigators found a very high accuracy in defining the exact TNM (>90%) when FDG-PET/CT was compared with conventional imaging results.

Apparently, the main drawback of FDG-PET/CT is the relatively reduced sensitivity for the detection of lung metastases, especially at the time of diagnosis. This reduced sensitivity is mainly caused by the spatial resolution of PET imaging, which conventionally is considered about 5 mm, preventing the visualization of initial tiny metastases. This lack of visualization can be overwhelmed by associating a diagnostic chest CT to the FDG-PET scan to correctly stage the disease.[12,13]

Charest and colleagues[13] retrospectively analyzed a series of 212 patients with known soft tissue or osseous sarcoma who had undergone a FDG-PET/CT study for the initial staging or assessment of recurrence of disease. FDG-PET/CT detected 93.9% of all sarcomas with a sensitivity of 93.7% for soft tissue sarcomas and 94.6% for osseous sarcomas. The sensitivities of the most common sarcoma histologies were 100% for leiomyosarcomas, 94.7% for osteosarcomas, 100% for Ewing sarcomas, 88.9% for liposarcomas, 80% for synovial sarcomas, 100% for GISTs, 87.5% for malignant peripheral nerve sheath tumors, 100% for fibroblastic and myoblastic sarcomas, and 100% for malignant fibrohistiocytic tumors.

The receiver-operating characteristic curve revealed an area of 94% under the curve for the discrimination of low-grade and high-grade sarcomas imaged for initial staging by FDG-PET/CT. The investigators concluded that the combined metabolic and morphologic information of FDG-PET/CT imaging allows high sensitivity for the detection of various sarcomas and accurate discrimination between newly diagnosed low-grade and high-grade sarcomas.[14]

In addition, sarcoma recurrence can be successfully and easily demonstrated with FDG-PET in pediatric patients, which was demonstrated by Arush and colleagues[14] on a series of 19 patients. FDG-PET/CT scans of these patients helped in the correct interpretation of conventional imaging findings, and otherwise unknown metastases in 2 patients were detected.

Murakami and colleagues[15] used FDG-PET/CT procedure during a follow-up of 8 patients affected

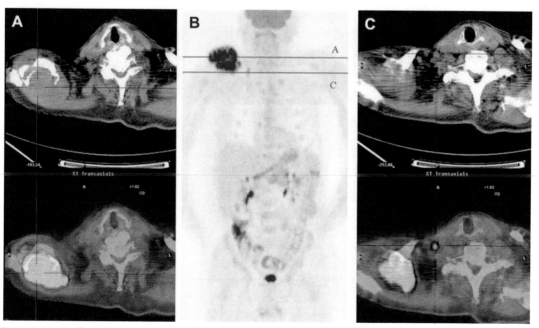

Fig. 3. Patient affected by a sarcoma of the soft tissues adjacent to the right clavicle. FDG-PET/CT was performed to stage the disease. (*A*) The primary tumor is detected. (*B*) Total body maximum intensity projection (MIP) image. (*C*) A secondary subcentrimetric supraclavicular lymph node is also detected.

by uterine sarcoma to highlight a disease recurrence. The patients also underwent US and CT, which had a lower detection rate compared with FDG-PET/CT. PET revealed recurrent sites in the intraperitoneum, liver, lung, bone, and retroperitoneal lymph nodes, whereas CT and US images showed 2 false-negative cases of intraperitoneal tumors. Positive PET findings helped to change patient management in 2 of 5 patients positive for recurrent sarcomas. The investigators concluded that the application of PET imaging for the early detection of recurrent sites was useful for deciding treatment strategy for patients with recurrent uterine sarcoma.

ONCOMING TRACERS

FDG was proved to be accurate and sensitive for the evaluation of soft tissue and bone sarcomas because the major components of these neoplastic diseases are intermediate- or high-grade tumors.

Some groups, however, tested different radiopharmaceuticals to understand if there may somehow be an added value in other tracers compared with FDG.

Buck and colleagues,[16] for example, evaluated the role of FLT-PET to differentiate benign from malignant tumors (FLT is a marker of proliferation) and to detect manifestation sites of bone and soft

tissue sarcomas. Their patient population consisted of 22 patients with established or suspected bone or soft tissue lesions. FLT-PET was compared with FDG-PET/CT, MR, CT, and biopsy. The investigators found a significant correlation between FLT uptake and tumor grade in biopsy, which was not found for FDG, and concluded that FLT-PET is a suitable imaging procedure to evaluate soft tissue and bone tumors.

Another interesting study by Tateishi and colleagues[17] is based on the use of choline-PET for staging 16 patients with soft tissue and bone sarcomas compared with bone scintigraphy, chest CT, and MR. In this case, tumor staging was confirmed by histologic examination and/or by an obvious progression in number and/or size of the lesions at follow-up examinations. The results were positive for PET because it gave a correct result for the assessment of TNM in 15 of 16 patients, whereas conventional imaging gave a correct result for TNM in 8 of 16 patients. The major limitation of this study, however, is the absence of data on FDG-PET/CT.

In addition, methionine was evaluated for the detection and assessment of neoadjuvant chemotherapy effect in combination with FDG in a preliminary study in 9 patients by Ghigi and colleagues.[18] This study demonstrated that, despite methionine's accuracy in highlighting the primary mass, FDG is more suitable for distinguishing responder

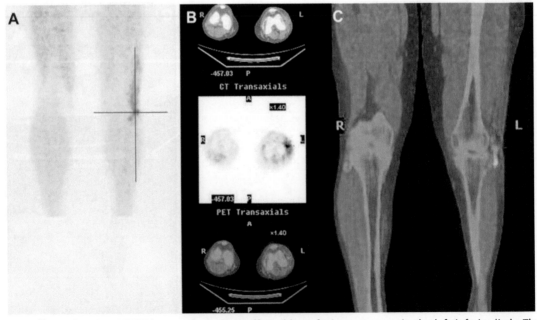

Fig. 4. [11]C methionine–PET/CT image of a patient affected by soft tissue sarcoma in the left inferior limb. The primary mass shows an increased uptake of tracer. (*A*) MIP image. (*B*) Axial views (CT, PET, fusion). (*C*) Sagittal view (fused CT and PET images).

from nonresponder patients, because the difference between pretherapy and posttherapy uptake is much greater for FDG in responder patients **(Fig. 4)**.

SUMMARY

According to the preliminary data published so far, PET seems to be a valuable method for evaluating patients with soft tissue and bone sarcomas. FDG seems to be the best tracer, but only a few articles are based on other compounds, therefore further studies are required before confirming this result.

FDG-PET/CT seems to be useful in predicting the patient prognosis, in assessing the response to neoadjuvant chemotherapy, and in staging or restaging the disease, significantly contributing to the correct management of the patient. Based on published data, it is possible to predict a future wider employment of this imaging method in patients affected by sarcomas.

REFERENCES

1. Skubitz KM, D'Adamo DR. Sarcoma [review]. Mayo Clin Proc 2007;82(11):1409–32.

2. Toner GC, Hicks RJ. PET for sarcomas other than gastrointestinal stromal tumors [review]. Oncologist 2008;13(Suppl 2):22–6.

3. Eary JF, O'Sullivan F, O'Sullivan J, et al. Spatial heterogeneity in sarcoma 18F-FDG uptake as a predictor of patient outcome. J Nucl Med 2008; 49(12):1973–9.

4. Lisle JW, Eary JF, O'Sullivan J, et al. Risk assessment based on FDG-PET imaging in patients with synovial sarcoma. Clin Orthop Relat Res 2009; 467(6):1605–11.

5. Punt SE, Eary JF, O'Sullivan J, et al. Fluorodeoxyglucose positron emission tomography in leiomyosarcoma: imaging characteristics. Nucl Med Commun 2009;30(7):546–9.

6. Evilevitch V, Weber WA, Tap WD, et al. Reduction of glucose metabolic activity is more accurate than change in size at predicting histopathologic response to neoadjuvant therapy in high-grade soft-tissue sarcomas. Clin Cancer Res 2008;14(3):715–20.

7. Shinto A, Nair N, Dutt A, et al. Early response assessment in gastrointestinal stromal tumors with FDG PET scan 24 hours after a single dose of imatinib. Clin Nucl Med 2008;33(7):486–7.

8. Prior JO, Montemurro M, Orcurto MV, et al. Early prediction of response to sunitinib after imatinib failure by 18F-fluorodeoxyglucose positron emission tomography in patients with gastrointestinal stromal tumor. J Clin Oncol 2009;27(3):439–45.

9. Benz MR, Evilevitch V, Allen-Auerbach MS, et al. Treatment monitoring by 18F-FDG PET/CT in patients with sarcomas: interobserver variability of quantitative parameters in treatment-induced changes in histopathologically responding and nonresponding tumors. J Nucl Med 2008;49(7): 1038–46.

10. Völker T, Denecke T, Steffen I, et al. Positron emission tomography for staging of pediatric sarcoma patients: results of a prospective multicenter trial. J Clin Oncol 2007;25(34):5435–41.

11. Tateishi U, Yamaguchi U, Seki K, et al. Bone and soft-tissue sarcoma: preoperative staging with fluorine 18 fluorodeoxyglucose PET/CT and conventional imaging. Radiology 2007;245(3):839–47.

12. Bestic JM, Peterson JJ, Bancroft LW. Use of FDG PET in staging, restaging, and assessment of therapy response in Ewing sarcoma. Radiographics 2009;29(5):1487–500.

13. Charest M, Hickeson M, Lisbona R, et al. FDG PET/CT imaging in primary osseous and soft tissue sarcomas: a retrospective review of 212 cases. Eur J Nucl Med Mol Imaging 2009;36:1944–51.

14. Arush MW, Israel O, Postovsky S, et al. Positron emission tomography/computed tomography with 18fluoro-deoxyglucose in the detection of local recurrence and distant metastases of pediatric sarcoma. Pediatr Blood Cancer 2007;49(7): 901–5.

15. Murakami M, Tsukada H, Shida M, et al. Whole-body positron emission tomography with F-18 fluorodeoxyglucose for the detection of recurrence in uterine sarcomas. Int J Gynecol Cancer 2006;16: 854–60.

16. Buck AK, Herrmann K, Büschenfelde CM, et al. Imaging bone and soft tissue tumors with the proliferation marker [18F]fluorodeoxythymidine. Clin Cancer Res 2008;14(10):2970–7.

17. Tateishi U, Yamaguchi U, Maeda T, et al. Staging performance of carbon-11 choline positron emission tomography/computed tomography in patients with bone and soft tissue sarcoma: comparison with conventional imaging. Cancer Sci 2006;97(10): 1125–8.

18. Ghigi G, Micera R, Maffione AM. 11C-Methionine vs 18F-FDG PET in soft tissue sarcoma patients treated with neoadjuvant therapy: preliminary results. In Vivo 2009;23(1):105–10.

^{18}F-Fluorodeoxy-glucose PET and PET/CT in Pediatric Musculoskeletal Malignancies

Frederick D. Grant, MD*, Laura A. Drubach, MD,
S. Ted Treves, MD

KEYWORDS

- FDG-PET • Pediatric tumors • Musculoskeletal tumors
- Osteosarcoma • Ewing sarcoma • Rhabdomyosarcoma

Musculoskeletal malignancies include a wide range of bone and soft-tissue tumors. Although uncommon, these tumors are major contributors to morbidity and mortality in children. Primary bone tumors are most prevalent in children and young adults, and include osteosarcoma and the Ewing family of tumors, which are the second and third most common solid tumors in children.[1] Patients of all ages, including children, can be affected by soft-tissue tumors, such as rhabdomyosarcoma and a wide variety of rare non-rhabdomyosarcoma soft-tissue malignancies.

Patient outcome depends on tumor type and grade, disease stage, and use of appropriate therapy. Imaging studies, including ^{18}F-fluorodeoxyglucose (FDG)-PET, play an important role in the planning and implementation of appropriate therapy. However, for most of these tumors the relative utility of different imaging modalities remains incompletely characterized. In pediatric patients, imaging frequently follows the practices used in adult patients, yet, even in adults, the appropriate use of techniques such as ^{18}F-FDG-PET remains unclear; this reflects that these tumors are uncommon, with few published studies using large numbers of well-characterized subjects. However, a thorough review of the available literature should help guide the appropriate use of ^{18}F-FDG-PET to evaluate musculoskeletal tumors in children and should identify specific needs for further investigation.

ROLE OF FDG-PET IN DIAGNOSIS

After identification of a musculoskeletal tumor, the first concern is distinguishing a benign tumor from malignancy. Although many bone and soft-tissue lesions have distinctive imaging appearances on radiography, computed tomography (CT), or magnetic resonance (MR) imaging, most will require further evaluation. Tissue sampling is almost always necessary to make a definitive diagnosis. Many investigators have studied the utility of ^{18}F-FDG-PET for distinguishing malignant tumors from benign processes. As there are few data available for pediatric musculoskeletal tumors, extrapolation must be made from studies including patients of all ages.

In general, malignant tumors demonstrate greater FDG avidity than benign lesions. However, it has been difficult to use this information for tumor diagnosis. In groups of adults and children with bone and soft-tissue tumors,[2,3] there was significant correlation between FDG uptake and

The authors have nothing to disclose.

Division of Nuclear Medicine and Molecular Imaging, Children's Hospital Boston, and the Joint Program in Nuclear Medicine, Harvard Medical School, 300 Longwood Avenue, Boston, MA 02115, USA

* Corresponding author.

E-mail address: frederick.grant@childrens.harvard.edu

PET Clin 5 (2010) 349–361

doi:10.1016/j.cpet.2010.05.001

tumor grade. However, FDG uptake could not distinguish benign lesions from low-grade malignant tumors. In another study of 45 patients of all ages, each patient had a diagnosis of either malignant or benign lesions in either bone or soft tissue.[4] Using a standardized uptake value (SUV) of 2.0 as a cut-off, ^{18}F-FDG-PET had an accuracy of 91.7% for distinguishing benign from malignant disease. Two malignant lesions had an SUV less than 2.0 and no benign lesions had an SUV greater than 2.0. Aoki and colleagues[5] also showed that malignant and benign lesions had significantly different FDG avidity, on average, but that there was too much overlap between the two groups to be clinically useful. This finding may, in part, reflect the difficulty in standardizing calculation of an SUV in a clinical environment.[6,7] In particular, FDG uptake in benign lesions has a broader distribution, which results in overlap with FDG uptake values in malignant lesions. For example, benign lesions containing giant cells or histiocytes can be FDG-avid, whereas chondrosarcoma can be non–FDG-avid.

Bischoff and colleagues[8] investigated the use of integrated PET/CT for diagnostic evaluation of bone and soft-tissue tumors. In a group of 80 patients with either malignant[9] or benign[10] tumors PET, CT, and PET/CT were all interpreted individually. Although, on average, malignant lesions had higher FDG uptake, overlap between benign and malignant lesions limited the use of FDG uptake to predict tumor grade.

Therefore, ^{18}F-FDG-PET, with or without concurrent conventional imaging, is not sufficiently accurate to serve as a noninvasive method of determining if a soft-tissue or bone lesion is benign or malignant. However, one potential diagnostic role for ^{18}F-FDG-PET/CT can be to guide diagnostic procedures, such as needle biopsy, to facilitate sampling of the most active region of a tumor.[11,12]

ROLE OF FDG-PET IN PATIENT MANAGEMENT

Once the diagnosis of musculoskeletal malignancy is known, ^{18}F-FDG-PET may have roles in staging disease, assessing the response to chemotherapy, and evaluating for disease recurrence. For most musculoskeletal tumors, successful treatment includes a combination of systemic chemotherapy and local control, which may be either surgery or radiation therapy. Disease management depends on disease stage, which requires accurate identification of all sites of disease. The use of neoadjuvant chemotherapy[13] may facilitate limb-sparing procedures and decrease the need for complete amputation. The histologic assessment of response to neoadjuvant therapy is prognostic and informs the planning of subsequent surgery. A noninvasive measure of tumor response to therapy, such as ^{18}F-FDG-PET, would be helpful in this planning. Finally, ^{18}F-FDG-PET may be helpful in the early detection of recurrent disease.

OSTEOSARCOMA
Clinical

Osteosarcoma is the most common bone tumor of children and young adults, and 80% of osteosarcomas present between ages of 5 and 25 years.[1] A second peak of incidence in older adults is much more likely to be secondary osteosarcoma. Primary osteosarcoma occurs predominately in the metaphyses of the long bones of the extremities, with less than one-third occurring in other locations. Secondary osteosarcoma occurs at the sites of other pathologic processes in bone, such as Paget disease, fibrous dysplasia, and multiple chondromas. The occurrence of osteosarcoma also is associated with retinoblastoma and prior radiation exposure. Osteosarcoma has a wide range of pathologic subtypes based on histologic characteristics and location in the body and bone. Over half the cases of osteosarcoma are found to have metastases at or soon after diagnosis. The most common site of metastatic disease is lung. Less commonly, 10% to 20% of metastases are in bone, but lymph node metastatic disease is rare.[14]

Before the introduction of effective chemotherapy, the 2-year survival rate for osteosarcoma was 20%. The combination of multiagent chemotherapy and local control has improved survival to 65% to 70% event-free survival in patients with localized disease.[15] Osteosarcoma is resistant to radiation therapy,[14] so that surgery is the only option for local control in these patients.

Local control is important to outcome; inadequate local control is associated with local treatment failure and poor outcome in osteosarcoma.[16,17] Secondary osteosarcoma has a worse prognosis than primary osteosarcoma.[14] Osteosarcoma therapy is dependent on staging.[18] Treatment of recurrent disease is important to survival, so it is imperative to find recurrent disease to improve survival. Surgical resection of metastases can improve survival by up to 50%.[18]

Diagnosis and Staging

^{18}F-FDG-PET has been used in the initial evaluation and staging of osteosarcoma (**Fig. 1**). FDG avidity, as measured by average SUV$_{max}$, is higher

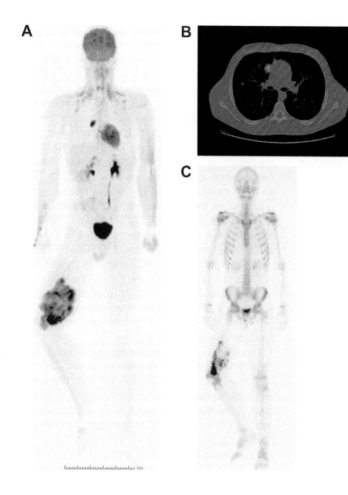

Fig. 1. ^{18}F-FDG-PET of osseous and pulmonary metastases in metastatic osteosarcoma. (*A*) A maximum-intensity projection (MIP) of an ^{18}F-FDG-PET scan performed in a 15 year-old boy with the new diagnosis of osteosarcoma demonstrates heterogeneous uptake in the large osseous and soft-tissue mass in the right thigh, chest, and in multiple left anterior ribs. (*B*) A transaxial CT fusion image demonstrates that focal chest uptake correlates with a large lung nodule in the right lung, adjacent to the mediastinum, while uptake is not seen in multiple smaller lung nodules. (*C*) ^{99m}Tc-MDP whole body bone scan shows heterogeneous uptake in the mass in the right femur, including uptake in some of the soft-tissue components of the tumor. No abnormal uptake is seen in the multiple pulmonary nodules or in the left anterior ribs, suggesting bone marrow disease without involvement of cortical bone. Although ^{99m}Tc-MDP bone scan typically has higher sensitivity than ^{18}F-FDG-PET for skeletal metastases, in some cases ^{18}F-FDG-PET may identify osseous metastases before a bone scan.

in osteosarcoma than in most other sarcomas.[19] Several investigators have attempted to use FDG uptake to assess tumor grade.[3,20] In children with osteosarcoma, low FDG uptake is associated with longer event-free and overall survival.[21] However, predicting tumor grade has been limited by heterogeneous uptake in the tumor mass, typically with more uptake in the periphery than in central regions.[20]

An early study demonstrated than ^{18}F-FDG could be used to identify osseous skip lesions.[22] However, definitive studies of the utility of ^{18}F-FDG for bone lesions have been limited by the small number of osseous metastases that occur with osteosarcoma.[23] Franzius and colleagues[24] compared ^{18}F-FDG-PET with planar ^{99m}Tc-methyldiphosphonate (^{99m}Tc-MDP) bone scan to detect osseous metastases of bone tumors, including 32 patients with osteosarcoma, 5 of whom had a bone metastasis. Although none of the bone metastases were identified by ^{18}F-FDG-PET, all 5 metastases were seen on bone scan. This result is consistent with the

osteoblastic characteristic of osteosarcoma.[24,25] One of the same research groups[26] showed that in a small number of osteosarcoma patients, whole body MR imaging could be better than whole body (head to feet)[18]F-FDG-PET, but MR imaging had no advantage over whole body bone scan. In contrast, Volker and colleagues[19] reported 90% sensitivity for ^{18}F-FDG-PET and only 81% for bone scan in identifying osseous metastases, but demonstrated 100% sensitivity when images from all modalities were compared in side-by-side analysis. The initial PET changed local control or systemic therapy in only 1 of 11 patients with osteosarcoma, but this is more a reflection of the current treatment strategy for osteosarcoma, in which initial staging does not determine the chemotherapy regimen.

Soon after the introduction of ^{18}F-FDG-PET into clinical use, it was used to identify metastatic lung lesions in patients with osteosarcoma. Identification of lung metastases is particularly important in the management of osteosarcoma, as lung metastases at the time of diagnosis makes 2-year survival unlikely, but surgical resection of all lung metastases can improve long-term survival to 20% to 50%. Early investigators reported that ^{18}F-FDG-PET and single detector CT had similar accuracy for finding lung metastases,[3,27] but later studies demonstrated spiral CT detected twice as many lung metastases as FDG-PET.[28] This improvement likely reflected the improvement in the sensitivity of CT with the introduction of spiral CT during this time. Although ^{18}F-FDG-PET was less sensitive than spiral CT, especially for lung lesions less than 9 mm in size, ^{18}F-FDG-PET and spiral CT showed similar high levels of specificity.[28]

There are few published data assessing the utility of ^{18}F-FDG-PET for finding the rare osteosarcoma metastases that occur at sites other than lungs or bones. Compared with regional CT studies, ^{18}F-FDG-PET has a larger field of view and a better opportunity to identify soft-tissue metastatic disease.

Response to Therapy

Response to neoadjuvant chemotherapy, with greater than 90% necrosis considered a favorable response, is associated with a much lower rate of local recurrence than occurs in tumors with an unfavorable response.[27] One study has reported that the response of osteosarcoma to neoadjuvant therapy predicts disease-free survival.[29] In addition to being a prognostic indicator, the response to neoadjuvant chemotherapy can guide the surgical approach,[30] and can help avoid further exposure to ineffective chemotherapy.[14]

Although FDG-PET may have a role in the preoperative assessment of the response to neoadjuvant chemotherapy, many different methods have been used for assessing FDG uptake. Some studies have demonstrated that a decrease of 30% to 40% in tumor-to-background ratio during therapy correlates with a favorable histologic response,[27,31,32] but in 2 studies, tumor uptake did not predict of the degree of tumor necrosis in any individual patient.[27,31] Other investigators have demonstrated that a 25% to 50% reduction in SUV$_{peak}$ uptake may better correlate with tumor necrosis, but these studies had false-positive findings due to benign processes, such as inflammation.[33,34] ^{18}F-FDG-PET performs better than bone scan in the preoperative assessment of osteosarcoma.[31] This lack of correlation between ^{18}F-FDG-PET and bone scan likely reflects a tendency of bone scan to overestimate the extent of disease[35] and the slower response of bone scan to the effects of therapy.

More recent studies[34,36] have shown that on the posttherapy, presurgical scan, the SUV$_{max}$ is the strongest predictor of histopathological response to neoadjuvant chemotherapy. FDG uptake on the preoperative study or a ratio of uptake posttherapy uptake to pretherapy uptake was only a moderate predictor of histologic response. A recent study by Cheon and colleagues[37] used receiver-operator characteristics (ROC) to develop models that used ^{18}F-FDG-PET and MR imaging for the preoperative prediction of the histopathological response to neoadjuvant chemotherapy. Overall, tumor SUV on the postchemotherapy study was a good predictor of tumor response, but was limited at intermediate levels of FDG uptake. Although change in tumor size as assessed by MR imaging alone was not better than ^{18}F-FDG-PET, the combination of change in tumor size by MR and FDG uptake by PET strengthened the ability of preoperative ^{18}F-FDG-PET to predict the tumor response to therapy. However, histopathological response still could not be predicted with intermediate levels of FDG uptake.

Therefore, for osteosarcoma, preoperative assessment of FDG uptake is a predictor of outcome and an indicator of the histologic response to neoadjuvant chemotherapy. Although many different measures of FDG uptake can be used, it seems that SUV$_{max}$, possibly in combination with tumor response on MR imaging, may be the most useful. However, in patients with intermediate levels of FDG uptake, it still may be difficult to predict the tumor response to therapy.

Recurrence

In a small study of 6 patients, ^{18}F-FDG-PET found all sites of local recurrence but also had 1 false-positive result.[23] Lucas and colleagues[3] compared the performance of MR imaging and ^{18}F-FDG-PET for imaging local disease. Although MR appeared to be more sensitive than FDG for identifying local recurrence, MR imaging was affected adversely by implant artifacts. In addition, whole body ^{18}F-FDG-PET found 13 other sites of metastatic recurrent disease that were outside the field of view of regional MR imaging.

One particular challenge in the management of musculoskeletal tumors is evaluation for recurrence in the stump at an amputation site. FDG uptake in the remaining bone of a stump has been reported for up to 18 months after surgery,[11] likely reflecting continued trauma from weight bearing with a prosthesis.[38] Thus, recurrence should be diagnosed with caution, while true recurrence could be obscured by inflammatory uptake at the stump.

EWING SARCOMA
Clinical

Ewing sarcoma is a tumor of the skeleton and adjacent soft tissue, and is the second most frequent bone tumor of children and young adults.[9] The Ewing family of tumors encompasses a histologically heterogeneous group of tumors, including sarcomas of bone, soft tissue, and nerves, including primitive neuroectodermal tumors (PNET). Ewing tumors can occur anywhere in the body. Metastatic disease is common; approximately one-quarter of patients have metastatic disease at diagnosis. Lung, bone, and bone marrow are the most common sites of metastases.[39] Metastatic relapse occurs in up to one-third of patients who had nonmetastatic disease at the time of diagnosis.[40]

The prognosis of Ewing tumors depends on the extent of disease and the use of appropriate therapy. The combination of multiagent chemotherapy and local control has improved survival to a 60% to 70% chance of event-free survival with localized disease.[15] Inadequate local control is associated with local treatment failure and poor outcome in Ewing sarcoma.[41] Distant disease is associated with even poorer survival. Long-term survival is only 40% for patients with lung metastases and less than 20% for patients with osseous metastases or bone marrow invasion.[15,40,42,43]

Diagnosis and Staging

The initial diagnosis of a Ewing tumor typically is made during assessment of symptoms, such as musculoskeletal pain, with radiographs or MR imaging (**Fig. 2**). For imaging the local primary disease site, the performance of ^{18}F-FDG-PET is no better than conventional imaging,[19] and tumor FDG avidity is not associated with prognosis in Ewing sarcoma.[10]

Identification of sites of disease and localization of metastases affects staging and initial risk stratification, but is particularly important for Ewing sarcoma, as all sites of disease receive local therapy.[9] MR imaging may be used to assess the local extent of disease, whereas the standard evaluation for distant disease has included bone scan, chest CT, and bone marrow aspiration. Whole body imaging, such as ^{18}F-FDG-PET or whole body MR imaging, may have a role in identifying distant sites of disease. Although both ^{18}F-FDG-PET and whole body MR imaging can identify soft-tissue disease, neither[28] is ideal for identifying lung metastases. In particular, CT is better than ^{18}F-FDG-PET for finding lung metastases less than 8 mm.[19] Therefore, a chest CT remains an essentially part of the staging process. Depending on the imaging protocol, an adequate chest CT may be available as part of a PET/CT study.

For identification of skeletal disease, both MR imaging and FDG-PET are more sensitive than ^{99m}Tc-MDP bone scan,[9,44] but ^{18}F-FDG-PET is more sensitive than whole body MR imaging.[26] This result is in concordance with another study[24] that showed ^{18}F-FDG-PET to perform better than planar bone scan in detecting osseous metastases in Ewing sarcoma. Specifically, whole body MR imaging is less sensitive than ^{18}F-FDG-PET in detecting disease in the ribs,[26] growth plates, and marrow.[45] These findings likely reflect that a bone scan images the osseous response to tumor, whereas ^{18}F-FDG-PET images the metabolic activity of the tumor regardless of cortical bone involvement. Thus, it may not be surprising that ^{18}F-FDG-PET is more sensitive than bone scan in detecting sites of Ewing sarcoma, which typically involves the bone marrow and is osteolytic.[24,25]

In one patient-based analysis of pediatric patients with Ewing sarcoma,[19] ^{18}F-FDG-PET was 91% accurate whereas conventional imaging was only 47% accurate in locating sites of distant disease, and ^{18}F-FDG-PET findings led to changes in local control or chemotherapy in approximately half of the patients. However, this study did not assess the effect of ^{18}F-FDG-PET on patient survival. Although ^{18}F-FDG-PET appears superior to either whole body ^{99m}Tc-MDP bone scan or MR imaging in patients with Ewing sarcoma, some comparative studies report lesions that are seen on bone scan but are not identified by either whole body MR imaging or ^{18}F-FDG-PET.[46] However, most comparisons between ^{18}F-FDG-PET and ^{99m}Tc-MDP bone scan use planar whole body bone scans, which may not be as sensitive as either a single-photon emission CT ^{99m}Tc-MDP bone scan or ^{18}F-NaF PET bone scan,[47] suggesting that the ideal approach to assessing patients with Ewing sarcoma for distant skeletal disease has not been resolved. Also unclear is whether the combination of FDG-PET and whole body bone scan to differentiate bone marrow disease from cortical bone involvement provides prognostic information.

Much less information is available regarding the use of ^{18}F-FDG-PET for assessment of PNET. One case report showed FDG avidity in a pelvic PNET,[48] while another case reported FDG avidity in a spinal PNET.[49]

Response to Therapy

For Ewing sarcoma, MR imaging typically has been used for assessment of the response of local

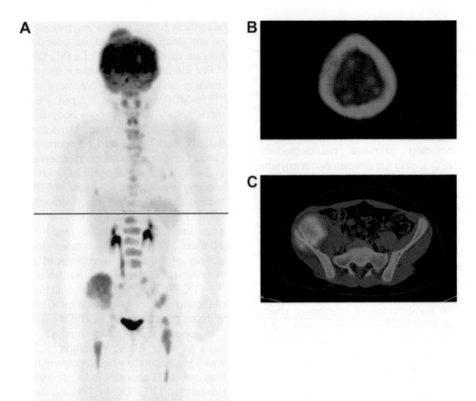

Fig. 2. ^{18}F-FDG-PET used to identify multiple sites of disease in metastatic Ewing sarcoma. An MIP of a staging ^{18}F-FDG-PET (*A*) and a contrast-enhanced CT scan in an 8-year-old girl with Ewing sarcoma demonstrate abnormal soft tissue in the head, pelvis, and axial skeleton. Transaxial PET and CT fusion images demonstrate mixed soft-tissue and osseous involvement in the right skull (*B*) and pelvis (*C*). Widespread FDG-avid metastatic skeletal disease is seen, including in the left sacrum (*C*). The wide field of view of PET facilitates identification of distant sites of disease.

disease. MR imaging still relies on size criteria and contrast enhancement, although enhancement is somewhat related to size, not viability.[50] MR imaging may not reliably distinguish vital tumor versus necrotic mass and has difficulty detecting minimal residual disease.[51] The ability to assess metabolic activity should allow FDG-PET to better assess response to therapy.[31] The European Organization for Research and Treatment of Cancer aimed to establish a standardized approach to assessing tumor response,[52] but this has not been widely implemented. Hawkins and colleagues[13] studied the role of FDG-PET in assessing response to therapy, suggesting that preoperative FDG avidity predicted histologic response to neoadjuvant chemotherapy. The same group later showed that, in patients with nonmetastatic Ewing sarcoma, decreased FDG uptake (SUV_{max} <2.5) after adjuvant chemotherapy predicted prolonged progression-free survival.[43]

With the availability of PET/CT, more recent studies have attempted to assess the utility of

FDG-PET/CT in assessing the response to therapy. Some of the earliest reports suggested a role for ^{18}F-FDG-PET/CT in assessing the response to therapy in a group of subjects with a wide variety of sarcomas.[53] As part of EURO-E.W.I.N.G. 99, Gerth and colleagues[54] reported on 53 subjects with Ewing sarcoma. The combination of ^{18}F-FDG-PET/CT performed with a low-dose CT plus a diagnostic lung CT outperformed ^{18}F-FDG-PET used alone. ^{18}F-FDG-PET/CT found new lesions not identified by FDG-PET, although most of the improvement in accuracy appeared driven by new lung metastases found on the diagnostic lung CT. The investigators did not report whether the low-dose CT performed as part of the PET/CT was sufficient to identify these lung metastases. PET/CT also identified additional bone lesions, although many of these proved to be benign. Overall, ^{18}F-FDG-PET/CT was reported to result in fewer equivocal lesions, and ^{18}F-FDG-PET/CT improved localization of disease, which could affect the approach to local control.

Recurrence

Very little has been published regarding the utility of ^{18}F-FDG-PET or ^{18}F-FDG-PET/CT for detection of local or distant recurrence of Ewing sarcoma. For detection of metastatic recurrence in the lung, CT performs better than PET.[3,28,55] In one study[46] of 9 pediatric patients with clinically suspected recurrent Ewing sarcoma, conventional imaging and ^{18}F-FDG-PET/CT identified recurrent disease in 5 subjects and confirmed the absence of recurrent disease in 4 subjects. In 1 subject with recurrent disease, PET did not detect a skull lesion detected by conventional bone scan. Therefore, ^{18}F-FDG-PET may have a role for identifying recurrent Ewing sarcoma, but the relative utility of ^{18}F-FDG-PET/CT, ^{99m}Tc-MDP bone scan, and other conventional imaging techniques remains unresolved.

RHABDOMYOSARCOMA
Clinical

Rhabdomyosarcoma is the most common malignant soft-tissue tumor affecting children and accounts for 4% to 8% cases of cancer in children younger than 15 years. About 350 new pediatric cases are diagnosed per year in the United States.[56] There are numerous histologic subtypes of rhabdomyosarcoma[57] and, in children, more than 70% of cases are embryonal subtype while approximately one-fifth of cases are alveolar subtype; other subtypes are rare. Unfortunately, published studies typically do not distinguish these subtypes when assessing the role of ^{18}F-FDG-PET in the evaluation of rhabdomyosarcoma. In over half of all cases of pediatric rhabdomyosarcoma, the primary site is in the skull or head and neck. The next most common primary site is the bladder or prostate. In less than 5% of cases, rhabdomyosarcoma presents as disseminated disease with an unknown primary.[58]

Therapy for rhabdomyosarcoma includes systemic multiagent chemotherapy combined with local control, which may be either surgery or radiation therapy.[59] Inadequate local control is associated with local treatment failure and poor outcome in patients with rhabdomyosarcoma.[57,60] Involvement of regional lymph nodes also is associated with poorer overall survival.[61]

Diagnosis and Staging

Improving the initial assessment of rhabdomyosarcoma with ^{18}F-FDG-PET can help patient management.[62] This assessment includes identification of regional adenopathy not seen on conventional imaging, which can affect the surgical approach for local control (**Fig. 3**). Identification of occult metastatic disease may guide decisions about local control and can lead to intensified chemotherapy. In addition, ^{18}F-FDG-PET may help to clarify ambiguous findings on conventional imaging studies.

In a study of pediatric musculoskeletal malignancies,[19] 12 subjects had rhabdomyosarcoma. ^{18}F-FDG-PET and conventional imaging performed equally in imaging the primary tumor, but ^{18}F-FDG-PET was better than conventional imaging for identifying lymph node involvement. In a patient-based analysis, ^{18}F-FDG-PET was 91% accurate and conventional imaging modalities were 47% accurate for identifying metastatic lymph node disease. ^{18}F-FDG-PET findings led to changes in local control or chemotherapy in approximately half the subjects with rhabdomyosarcoma.

In a study with 28 subjects with childhood rhabdomyosarcoma,[53] ^{18}F-FDG-PET/CT was sensitive for lymph node disease when used for initial staging. In another study,[62] 24 subjects with rhabdomyosarcoma were imaged with ^{18}F-FDG-PET/CT. These subjects were atypical, as 14 cases were alveolar subtype and only 10 were embryonal subtype. Of 96 lesions identified on the 24 initial ^{18}F-FDG-PET/CT studies, biopsy was used for confirmation of metastatic disease in only 7. Of 21 sites that were not identified on either CT or MR imaging, 19 were confirmed by PET, with only 1 false-positive finding on ^{18}F-FDG-PET. Some of the lymph nodes identified only by ^{18}F-FDG-PET later became positive on examination or by conventional imaging. Of 23 ambiguous sites on conventional imaging, 21 were excluded by ^{18}F-FDG-PET, which demonstrates another potential role for ^{18}F-FDG-PET. Ten sites identified by conventional imaging, but missed by FDG-PET, either were adjacent to a hot primary or appeared very small on conventional imaging. However, in none of the lesions was biopsy performed to confirm disease. Therefore, ^{18}F-FDG-PET appeared to have 64% sensitivity regional lymph node disease (although the sensitivity was 100% for lymph nodes that were biopsied), and the investigators concluded that ^{18}F-FDG-PET cannot replace biopsy for suspicious lymph nodes.

These findings suggest that, in the management of rhabdomyosarcoma, two roles for ^{18}F-FDG-PET are earlier identification of lymph node disease and excluding disease at sites of ambiguous findings on conventional imaging. ^{18}F-FDG-PET can also be useful to detect widespread bone marrow involvement.[63] Approximately 4% of cases of rhabdomyosarcoma present as disseminated disease with an unknown primary. In these patients, ^{18}F-FDG-PET/CT can be helpful in

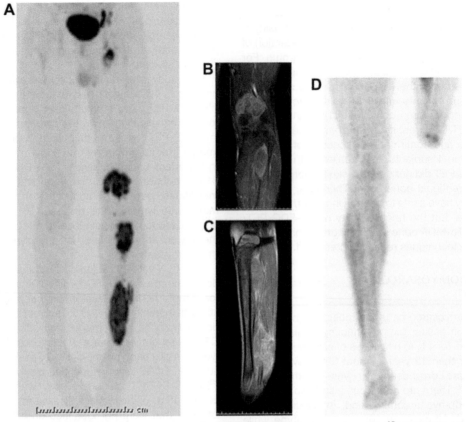

Fig. 3. Staging and assessment for recurrence of multifocal rhabdomyosarcoma with ^{18}F-FDG-PET. (*A*) MIP of a staging ^{18}F-FDG-PET in a 16-year-old boy presenting with multifocal alveolar rhabdomyosarcoma shows intense uptake in 3 leg lesions that correspond to soft-tissue masses identified with contrast-enhanced MR imaging (*B, C*) and in the left inguinal region. Biopsy demonstrated metastatic disease in an inguinal lymph node, demonstrating the value the wide field of view of ^{18}F-FDG-PET. (*D*) MIP of a follow-up ^{18}F-FDG-PET scan performed 4 years after multimodality therapy, including surgical amputation, shows no FDG-avid disease. Stable mild uptake in the stump of the left leg is related to weight bearing.

finding the primary due to its wide field of view (up to the whole body) and high sensitivity with specificity.

Response to Therapy

Very little has been reported about the use of ^{18}F-FDG-PET or ^{18}F-FDG-PET/CT in assessing the response of rhabdomyosarcoma to therapy. Bredella and colleagues[64] used ^{18}F-FDG-PET and MR to assess the response to therapy for a variety of tumors, although MR was limited by metal artifact. Only 2 of the 12 subjects had pediatric rhabdomyosarcoma. In one case, a residual mass with SUV 2.8 contained tumor at the time of resection, whereas in a mass with SUV 1.6 no residual tumor was found. This result suggests that, as with other pediatric musculoskeletal tumors, ^{18}F-FDG-PET could assess the response to therapy for pediatric

rhabdomyosarcoma, but larger patient series will be needed to confirm this role of FDG-PET.

Recurrence

In patients presenting with nonmetastatic rhabdomyosarcoma, local recurrence accounts for 85% of the treatment failures,[60] while the remainder of disease recurrence is at distant sites. There is little published research describing the role of ^{18}F-FDG-PET in identifying recurrent rhabdomyosarcoma. In one study[46] including 6 patients evaluated for recurrent rhabdomyosarcoma, the accuracy of all imaging studies for detecting local recurrence was limited by postsurgical changes, although in one case ^{18}F-FDG-PET/CT was useful to exclude local recurrent disease. ^{18}F-FDG-PET/CT was the only modality identifying distant disease in 2 subjects, but in a third subject ^{18}F-FDG-PET/CT missed a site of metastatic disease in a cervical lymph node. One limitation of this small study was that it did not clearly specify whether the CT was acquired only as part of the PET/CT or if a separate diagnostic CT scan was performed.

As with other musculoskeletal tumors, CT is more accurate than ^{18}F-FDG-PET in identifying lung metastases.[3,28,46,55] In a study of 35 patients with rhabdomyosarcoma,[65] ^{18}F-FDG-PET/CT was compared with conventional imaging, including ^{99m}Tc-MDP bone scan, CT, and MR imaging. ^{18}F-FDG-PET/CT and conventional imaging performed similarly in identifying the primary tumor and local lymph node involvement. ^{18}F-FDG-PET/CT was more accurate (89%) than conventional imaging (54% accurate) for distant metastases. ^{18}F-FDG-PET/CT was particularly useful in detecting recurrence of alveolar rhabdomyosarcoma, which can metastasize to unusual soft-tissue sites such as the pancreas and breast.

NON-RHABDOMYOSARCOMA SARCOMAS
Clinical

The category of non-rhabdomyosarcoma sarcomas includes a heterogeneous group of rare tumors, the most common of which include synovial cell sarcoma, malignant fibrous histiocytoma, fibrosarcoma, chondrosarcoma, angiosarcoma, and leiomyosarcoma in children.[1] Specific details of therapy can vary among the different histologic types but, as with the more common musculoskeletal tumors, the treatment depends on the principles of local control and systemic chemotherapy.

Use of ^{18}F-FDG-PET

Because non-rhabdomyosarcoma sarcomas are rare, there are no large clinical studies investigating the role of ^{18}F-FDG-PET in the diagnosis or staging of these tumors. Although many of the reports describing the use of ^{18}F-FDG-PET involve only adults, these tumors are included in larger series of pediatric tumors that include a variety of tumors, and there are reports describing the use of ^{18}F-FDG-PET or ^{18}F-FDG-PET/CT to assess one of these tumors in a single or small number of patients (**Fig. 4**). For example, these reports include cases demonstrating the use of FDG-PET in the management of synovial cell sarcoma,[66–68] angiosarcoma,[69] and malignant peripheral nerve sheath tumors[70] in pediatric patients. Therefore, the use of ^{18}F-FDG-PET to

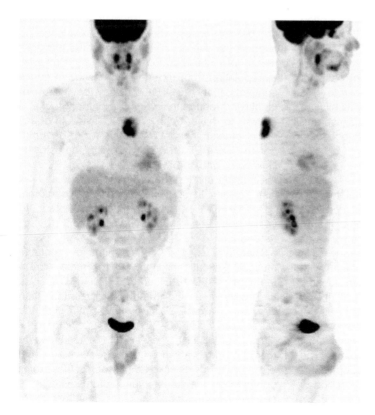

Fig. 4. ^{18}F-FDG-PET used to evaluate a non-rhabdomyosarcoma sarcoma. ^{18}F-FDG-PET was used to evaluate a 16-year-old boy with recurrent leiomyosarcoma in the mid-back. The recurrent tumor is intensely FDG-avid with no other sites of FDG-avid disease. In patients with non-rhabdomyosarcoma sarcoma, ^{18}F-FDG-PET is most useful to assess for recurrent or metastatic disease if the FDG avidity of the primary tumor is known.

evaluate these tumors must be done on a case-by-case basis. Better understanding of the utility of ^{18}F-FDG-PET likely will require multi-institutional studies performed over a period of time.

LYMPHOMA

Although both Hodgkin disease and non-Hodgkin lymphoma are systemic diseases, in less than 5% of patients the primary, and sometimes only, site of disease is in the skeleton.[71] Identifying and assessing skeletal involvement is particularly challenging with this group of diseases. In a meta-analysis of 13 studies,[72] ^{18}F-FDG-PET had 54% sensitivity and 92% specificity for lymphoma involvement in bone marrow. Sensitivity was better with Hodgkin disease, and may be most useful for localization of a biopsy site, particularly if prior biopsies have been negative.

^{18}F-FDG-PET also may have a role to assess residual space-occupying lesions in the marrow at the end of treatment. Marrow lesions may be seen in up to two-thirds of patients at completion of therapy, but anatomic imaging modalities typically cannot distinguish residual disease from fibrosis at the sites of successfully treated disease.[73] ^{18}F-FDG-PET provides an effective method to distinguish active disease from inactive fibrosis,[74] with up to a 95% positive predictive value.[75] Although the time course of the resolution of FDG avidity in skeletal lymphoma has not been well studied, Weber[76] suggests that the performance of ^{18}F-FDG-PET may be best 4 to 6 weeks after completion of therapy. Although the use of ^{18}F-FDG-PET for detection of recurrent osseous lymphoma has not been studied, the role ^{18}F-FDG-PET or ^{18}F-FDG-PET/CT may be similar to that for the management of Hodgkin disease and non-Hodgkin lymphoma in more typical locations.

SUMMARY

In the initial staging of musculoskeletal tumors, ^{18}F-FDG-PET is useful for identifying and localizing sites of distant disease. In Ewing sarcoma, identifying sites of distant disease is important, as all sites of disease may receive local therapy such as surgery or radiation therapy. In patients with rhabdomyosarcoma, ^{18}F-FDG-PET can identify disease in distant lymph nodes and soft tissue, and can change disease management in half of the patients. In osteosarcoma, the most common sites of metastatic disease are bone and lungs, so that bone scan and chest CT cannot be replaced by ^{18}F-FDG-PET. Non-rhabdomyosarcoma sarcomas are rare, and with little reported experience the use of FDG-PET must be on a case-by-case basis. In osseous lymphoma, ^{18}F-FDG-PET is useful for identifying other sites of disease but also may help identify a site for diagnostic biopsy.

The response to neoadjuvant therapy as assessed by FDG uptake may help predict long-term prognosis in patients with osteosarcoma and Ewing sarcoma. However, it is more difficult to use ^{18}F-FDG-PET to guide changes in patient management. The response, as assessed by FDG, can help guide the surgical approach to local control and may guide changes in chemotherapy in nonresponsive patients. This approach is limited when there is an intermediate level of FDG uptake that cannot be categorized as indicating either a favorable or unfavorable response. Therefore, it seems most appropriate that the use of ^{18}F-FDG-PET to assess the response to neoadjuvant chemotherapy be within a clinical trial. One exception may be in patients who have been treated for osseous lymphoma, in whom ^{18}F-FDG-PET is helpful in distinguishing persistent disease from marrow fibrosis.

The use of ^{18}F-FDG-PET or ^{18}F-FDG-PET/CT to identify local recurrence of musculoskeletal malignancy has not been clearly established. However, the real strength of ^{18}F-FDG-PET is the whole body coverage that can be helpful for identifying sites of distant metastatic disease, particularly with the diagnoses of Ewing sarcoma and rhabdomyosarcoma. Because of the smaller number of cases, there is less evidence to support the use of ^{18}F-FDG-PET in the management of non-rhabdomyosarcoma. However, extrapolation from reported experience in adults suggests that ^{18}F-FDG-PET may be useful for identifying recurrence when the primary tumor is known to have been ^{18}F-FDG–avid. In many earlier studies, chest CT was shown to be superior to FDG-PET in identifying lung metastases. However, with the widespread use of PET/CT, the relative utility of an independent chest CT is less clear. In patients with osteosarcoma, ^{18}F-FDG-PET/CT may be complementary to whole body bone scan in finding sites of disease recurrence.

Therefore, in the management of pediatric musculoskeletal malignancies, the main advantages of ^{18}F-FDG-PET and ^{18}F-FDG-PET/CT are the ability to assess tumor activity, rather than size, and a large field of view that can include the whole body. ^{18}F-FDG-PET can be useful for initial staging of disease, assessing the response to therapy, and evaluating for disease recurrence, but the value of ^{18}F-FDG-PET in each of these roles depends on the tumor type. Future research is needed to better define the complementary use of

18F-FDG-PET/CT with other imaging studies such as 99mTc-MDP bone scan or chest CT in patients with pediatric musculoskeletal malignancies.

REFERENCES

1. Gurney JG, Swensen AR, Bulterys M. Malignant bone tumors. In: Ries LA, Smith MA, Gurney JG, et al, editors. NIH Pub. No. 99–4649. Cancer incidence and survival among children and adolescents: United States SEER Program 1975–1995. Bethesda (MD): National Cancer Institute, SEER Program; 1999.

2. Schuetze SM. Utility of positron emission tomography in sarcomas. Curr Opin Oncol 2006;18: 369–73.

3. Lucas JD, O'Doherty MJ, Cronin BF, et al. Prospective evaluation of soft tissue masses and sarcomas using fluorodeoxyglucose positron emission tomography. Br J Surg 1999;86:550–6.

4. Feldman F, van Heertum R, Manos C. 18FDG PET scanning of benign and malignant musculoskeletal lesions. Skeletal Radiol 2003;32:201–8.

5. Aoki J, Watanabe H, Shinozaki T, et al. FDG PET of primary benign and malignant bone tumors: standardized uptake value in 52 lesions. Radiology 2001;219:774–7.

6. Westerterp M, Pruim J, Oyen W, et al. Quantification of FDG PET studies using standardised uptake values in multi-centre trials: effects of image reconstruction, resolution and ROI definition parameters. Eur J Nucl Med Mol Imaging 2007;34:392–404.

7. Wahl RL, Jacene H, Kasamon Y, et al. From RECIST to PERCIST: Evolving considerations for PET response criteria in solid tumors. J Nucl Med 2009; 50(Suppl 1):122S–50S.

8. Bischoff M, Bischoff G, Buck A, et al. Integrated FDG-PET-CT: its role in the assessment of bone and soft tissue tumors. Arch Orthop Trauma Surg 2009. [Epub ahead of print].

9. Furth C, Amthauer H, Denecke T, et al. Impact of whole-body MRI and FDG-PET on staging and assessment of therapy response in a patient with Ewing sarcoma. Pediatr Blood Cancer 2006;47:607–11.

10. Hawkins DS, Schuetze SM, Butrynski JE, et al. [18F]Fluorodeoxyglucose positron emission tomography predicts outcome for Ewing sarcoma family of tumors. J Clin Oncol 2005;23:8828–34.

11. Jadvar H, Gamie S, Ramanna L, et al. Musculoskeletal system. Semin Nucl Med 2004;34:254–61.

12. Klaeser B, Mueller MD, Schmid RA, et al. PET-CT-guided interventions in the management of FDG-positive lesions in patients suffering from solid malignancies: initial experiences. Eur Radiol 2009; 19:1780–5.

13. Hawkins DS, Rajendran JG, Conrad EU III, et al. Evaluation of chemotherapy response in pediatric bone sarcomas by [F-18]-fluorodeoxy-D-glucose positron emission tomography. Cancer 2002;94: 3277–84.

14. Brenner W, Bohuslavizki KH, Eary JF. PET imaging of osteosarcoma. J Nucl Med 2003;44:930–42.

15. Grier HE, Krailo MD, Tarbell NJ, et al. Addition of ifosfamide and etoposide to standard chemotherapy for Ewing's sarcoma and primitive neuroectodermal tumor of bone. N Engl J Med 2003;348:694–701.

16. Bacci G, Briccoli A, Ferrari S, et al. Neoadjuvant chemotherapy for osteosarcoma of the extremity: long-term results of the Rozzoli's 4th protocol. Eur J Cancer 2001;37:2030–9.

17. Weeden S, Grimer RJ, Cannon SR, et al. The effect of local recurrence on survival in resected osteosarcoma. Eur J Cancer 2001;37:39–46.

18. Enneking WF. A system of staging musculoskeletal neoplasms. Clin Orthop Relat Res 1986;204:9–24.

19. Volker T, Denecke T, Steffen I, et al. Positron emission tomography for staging of pediatric sarcoma patients: results of a prospective multicenter trial. J Clin Oncol 2007;25:5435–41.

20. Eary JF, Conrad EU, Bruckner JD, et al. Quantitative [F-18] fluorodeoxyglucose positron emission tomography in pretreatment and grading of sarcoma. Clin Cancer Res 1998;4:1215–20.

21. Franzius C, Bielack S, Flege S, et al. Prognostic significance of 18F-FDG and 99mTc-methylene diphosphonate uptake in primary osteosarcoma. J Nucl Med 2002;43:1012–7.

22. Wuisman P, Enneking WF. Prognosis for patients who have osteosarcoma with skip metastases. J Bone Joint Surg Am 1990;72:60–8.

23. Franzius C, Daldrup-Link HE, Wagner-Bohn A, et al. FDG-PET for detection of recurrences from malignant primary bone tumors: comparison with conventional imaging. Ann Oncol 2002;13:157–60.

24. Franzius C, Sciuk J, Daldrup-Link HE, et al. FDG-PET for detection of osseous metastases from malignant primary bone tumours: comparison with bone scintigraphy. Eur J Nucl Med 2000;27:1305–11.

25. Reddick RL, Michelitch HJ, Levine AM, et al. Osteogenic sarcoma: a study of the ultrastructure. Cancer 1980;45:64–71.

26. Daldrup-Link HE, Franzius C, Link TM, et al. Whole-body MR imaging for detection of bone metastases in children and young adults: comparison with skeletal scintigraphy and FDG PET. Am J Radiol 2001; 177:229–36.

27. Schulte M, Brecht-Krauss D, Werner M, et al. Evaluation of neoadjuvant therapy response of osteogenic sarcoma using FDG PET. J Nucl Med 1999; 40:1637–43.

28. Franzius C, Daldrup-Link HE, Sciuk J, et al. FDG-PET for detection of pulmonary metastases from malignant primary bone tumors: comparison with spiral CT. Ann Oncol 2001;12:479–86.

29. Bielack SS, Kempf-Bielack B, Delling G, et al. Prognostic factors in high-grade osteosarcoma of the extremities or trunk: an analysis of 1,702 patients treated on neoadjuvant cooperative osteosarcoma study group protocols. J Clin Oncol 2002;20:776–90.

30. Schulte M, Brecht-Kraus D, Heymer B, et al. Grading of tumors and tumorlike lesions of bone: evaluation by FDG PET. J Nucl Med 2000;41:1695–701.

31. Franzius C, Sciuk J, Brinkschmidt C, et al. Evaluation of chemotherapy response in primary bone tumor with F-18 FDG positron emission tomography compared with histologically assessed tumor necrosis. Clin Nucl Med 2000;25:874–81.

32. Ye Z, Zhu J, Tian M, et al. Response of osteogenic sarcoma to neoadjuvant therapy: evaluated by ^{18}F-FDG-PET. Ann Nucl Med 2008;22:475–80.

33. Jones DN, McCowage GB, Sostman HD, et al. Monitoring of neoadjuvant therapy response of soft-tissue and musculoskeletal sarcoma using fluorine-18-FDG PET. J Nucl Med 1996;37:1438–44.

34. Hawkins DS, Conrad EU III, Butrynski JE, et al. [F-18]-Fluorodeoxy-D-glucose positron emission tomography response is associated with outcome for extremity osteosarcoma in children and young adults. Cancer 2009;115:3519–25.

35. Chew FS, Hudson TM. Radionuclide bone scanning of osteosarcoma: falsely extended uptake patterns. Am J Roentgenol 1982;139:49–54.

36. Hamada K, Tomita Y, Inoue A, et al. Evaluation of chemotherapy response in osteosarcoma with FDG-PET. Ann Nucl Med 2009;23:89095.

37. Cheon GJ, KLim MS, Lee JA, et al. Prediction model of chemotherapy response in osteosarcoma by ^{18}F-FDG PET and MRI. J Nucl Med 2009;50:1435–40.

38. Hain SF, O'Doherty MJ, Lucas JD, et al. ^{18}F-FDG PET in the evaluation of stumps following amputation for soft tissue sarcoma. Nucl Med Commun 1999;20:490.

39. Marec-Berard P, Philip T. Ewing sarcoma: the pediatrician's point of view. Pediatr Blood Cancer 2004;42:477–80.

40. Paulussen M, Ahrens S, Dunst J, et al. Localized Ewing tumor of the bone: final results of the cooperative Ewing's sarcoma study CESS 86. J Clin Oncol 2001;19:1818–29.

41. Krasin MJ, Rodriguez-Galindo C, Billups CA, et al. Definitive irradiation in multidisciplinary management of localized Ewing sarcoma family of tumors in pediatric patients: outcome and prognostic factors. Int J Radiat Oncol Biol Phys 2004;60:830–8.

42. Coterill SJ, Ahrens S, Paulussen M, et al. Prognostic factors in Ewing's tumor of bone: analysis of 975 patients from the European intergroup cooperative Ewing's sarcoma study group. J Clin Oncol 2000;18:3108–14.

43. Barker LM, Pendergrass TW, Sanders JE, et al. Survival after recurrence of Ewing's sarcoma family of tumors. J Clin Oncol 2005;23:4354–62.

44. Mazumdar A, Siegel MJ, Narra V, et al. Whole-body fast inversion recovery MR imaging of small cell neoplasms in pediatric patients: a pilot study. Am J Radiol 2002;179:1261–6.

45. Mentzel H-J, Kentouche K, Sauner C, et al. Comparison of whole-body STIR-MRI and ^{99m}Tc-methylene-diphosphonate scintigraphy in children with suspected multifocal bone lesions. Eur Radiol 2004;14:2297–302.

46. Weyl Ben AM, Israel O, Postovksy S, et al. Positron emission tomography/computed tomography with [18]Fluor-deoxyglucose in the detection of local recurrence and distant metastases of pediatric sarcoma. Pediatr Blood Cancer 2007;49:901–5.

47. Grant FD, Fahey FH, Packard AB, et al. Skeletal PET with ^{18}F-fluoride: applying new technology to an old tracer. J Nucl Med 2008;49:68–78.

48. Watanabe H, Kawano M, Takada M, et al. F-18 FDG PET imaging in a primitive neuroectodermal tumor. Clin Nucl Med 2006;31:484–5.

49. Meltzer CC, Townsend DW, Kottapally S, et al. FDG imaging of spinal cord primitive neuroectodermal tumor. J Nucl Med 1998;39:1207–9.

50. van der Woude HJ, Bloem JL, Hogendoorn PC. Preoperative evaluation and monitoring chemotherapy in patients with high-grade osteogenic and Ewing's sarcoma: review of current imaging modalities. Skeletal Radiol 1998;27:57–71.

51. MacVicar AD, Offiff JFC, Pringle J, et al. Ewing sarcoma: MR imaging of chemotherapy-induced changes with histologic correlation. Radiology 1992;184:859–64.

52. Young H, Baum R, Cremerius U, et al. Measurement of clinical and subclinical tumour response using [18F]-fluorodeoxyglucose and positron emission tomography: review and 1999 EORTC recommendations. Eur J Cancer 1999;35:1773–82.

53. McCarville MB, Christie R, Daw NJ, et al. PET/CT in the evaluation of childhood sarcomas. Am J Radiol 2004;184:1293–304.

54. Gerth HU, Juergens KU, Dirksen U, et al. Significant benefit of multimodal imaging: PET/CT compared with PET alone in staging and follow-up of patients with Ewing tumors. J Nucl Med 2007;48:1932–9.

55. Reboul-Marty J, Quintana E, Mosseri V, et al. Prognostic factors of alveolar rhabdomyosarcoma of childhood: an International Society of pediatric oncology study. Cancer 1991;68:493–8.

56. Raney RB, Anderson JR, Barr FG, et al. Rhabdomyosarcoma and undifferentiated sarcoma in the first two decades of life: a selective review of intergroup Rhabdomyosarcoma study group experience and rationale for intergroup Rhabdomyosarcoma study V. J Pediatr Hematol Oncol 2001;23:215–20.

57. Wharam MD, Meza J, Anderson J, et al. Failure pattern and factors predictive of local failure in rhabdomyosarcoma: a report of group III patients on the third intergroup rhabdomyosarcoma study. J Clin Oncol 2004;22:1902–8.

58. Etcubanas E, Pieper S, Stass S, et al. Rhabdomyosarcoma presenting as disseminated malignancy from an unknown primary site: a retrospective study of ten pediatric cases. Med Pediatr Oncol 1989;17: 39–44.

59. Baker KS, Anderson JR, Link H, et al. Benefit of intensified therapy for patients with local or regional embryonal rhabdomyosarcoma: results from the Intergroup Rhabdomyosarcoma Study IV. J Clin Oncol 2000;18:2427–34.

60. Flamant F, Rodary C, Rey A, et al. Treatment of non-metastatic rhabdomyosarcomas in childhood and adolescence. Results of the second study of the international society of paediatric oncology: MMT84. Eur J Cancer 1998;34:1050–62.

61. LaQuaglia MP. Extremity rhabdomyosarcoma: biological principles, staging, and treatment. Semin Surg Oncol 1993;9:510–9.

62. Klem ML, Grewal RK, Wexler LH, et al. PET for staging in rhabdomyosarcoma: an evaluation of PET as an adjunct to current staging tools. J Pediatr Hematol Oncol 2007;29:9–14.

63. Seshadri N, Wright P, Balan KK. Rhabdomyosarcoma with widespread bone marrow infiltration: beneficial management role for F-18 FDG PET. Clin Nucl Med 2007;32:787–9.

64. Bredella MA, Caputo GR, Steinbach LS. Value of FDG positron emission tomography in conjunction with MR imaging for evaluating therapy response in patients with musculoskeletal sarcomas. Am J Radiol 2002;179:1145–50.

65. Tateishi U, Hosono A, Makimoto A, et al. Comparative study of FDG PET/CT and conventional imaging in the staging of rhabdomyosarcoma. Ann Nucl Med 2009;23:155–61.

66. Kleis M, Daldrup-Link H, Matthay K, et al. Diagnostic value of PET/CT for the staging and restaging of pediatric tumors. Eur J Nucl Med Mol Imaging 2009;36:23–36.

67. Charest M, Hickeson M, Lisbona R, et al. FDG PET/CT imaging in primary osseous and soft tissue sarcomas: a retrospective review of 212 cases. Eur J Nucl Med Mol Imaging 2009;36:1944–51.

68. Lisle JW, Eary JF, O'Sullivan J, et al. Risk assessment based on FDG-PET imaging in patients with synovial sarcoma. Clin Orthop Relat Res 2009;467: 1605–11.

69. Zeng W, Styblo TM, Shiyong L, et al. Breast angiosarcoma: FDG PET findings. Clin Nucl Med 2009; 34:443–5.

70. Warbey VS, Ferner RE, Dunn JT, et al. [18F]FDG PET/CT in the diagnosis of malignant peripheral nerve sheath tumors in neurofibromatosis type-1. Eur J Nucl Med Mol Imaging 2009;36:751–7.

71. Furman WL, Fitch S, Hustu HO, et al. Primary lymphoma of bone in children. J Clin Oncol 1989; 7:1275–80.

72. Pakos EE, Fotopoulos AD, Ioannidis JPA. 18F-FDG PET for evaluation of bone marrow infiltration in staging of lymphoma: a meta-analysis. J Nucl Med 2005;46:958–63.

73. Duet M, Pouchet J, Liote F, et al. Role for positron emission tomography in skeletal diseases. Joint Bone Spine 2007;74:14–23.

74. Reske SN. PET and restaging of malignant lymphoma including residual masses and relapse. Eur J Nucl Med Mol Imaging 2003;30(Suppl 1): S89–96.

75. Castellucci P, Zinzani PL, Pourdehnad M, et al. 18F-FDG PET in malignant lymphoma: significance of positive findings. Eur J Nucl Med Mol Imaging 2005;32:749–56.

76. Weber WA. Use of PET for monitoring cancer therapy and for predicting outcome. J Nucl Med 2005;46:983–95.

Alternative PET Tracers in Musculoskeletal Disease

Akram Al-Ibraheem, MD, FEBNM[a], Andreas K. Buck, MD[b],
Ambros J. Beer, MD[b], Ken Herrmann, MD[b],*

KEYWORDS

- Musculoskeletal tumors • Detection
- Positron emission tomography • Radiolabeled tracers

Musculoskeletal tumors comprise a multitude of entities with different grades of malignancy, biologic behavior, and therapeutic options. The incidence is relatively low, and malignant tumors account for approximately 0.6% of all cancers.[1] In clinical practice, evaluation of many musculoskeletal lesions remains a diagnostic dilemma. In general, computed tomography (CT) and magnetic resonance (MR) imaging are excellent tools for visualizing anatomic details including location, extent, and inhomogeneity of a lesion. However, these noninvasive modalities are not sufficiently reliable indicators of the active tumor cell compartment or malignant potential.[2,3] Such information is crucial for preoperative planning, including selection of the initial surgical procedure and identification of metabolically active areas within the tumor to further assist in guiding biopsy.

PET allows noninvasive assessment of cancer biology and aids in the detection and staging of malignant tumors, detection of relapse, differentiating scar from residual active disease, or grading of tumors. PET using the glucose analog [18F]fluorodeoxyglucose (FDG) is now an established imaging modality for detection and staging of cancer.[4] Numerous studies have evaluated the role of imaging musculoskeletal tumors with FDG-PET. The literature has been comprehensively reviewed and analyzed by Bastiaannet and colleagues.[5] FDG-PET has the potential to discriminate between high-grade sarcomas and benign tumors, and between low- and high-grade malignant tumors based on the mean standardized uptake value (SUV). However, FDG-PET cannot be regarded as a standard method for differential diagnosis of musculoskeletal lesions. False-positive PET findings were reported in aggressive benign tumors and inflammatory lesions.[6–8] FDG is also inadequate to differentiate low-grade malignant lesions and benign tumors.[9]

The use of more specific radiopharmaceuticals such as the proliferation marker [18F]fluorodeoxythymidine (FLT), the bone-imaging agent [18F]fluoride, amino acid tracers ([11C]methionine, [18F]fluoroethyltyrosine) or biomarkers of neoangiogenesis ([18F]galacto-RGD) have been investigated to overcome some of these shortcomings and to provide insights into the biology of musculoskeletal tumors with a focus on tumor grading, treatment monitoring, posttherapy assessment, and estimation of individual prognosis. In this article, the potential role of these alternative PET tracers in musculoskeletal disorders is reviewed with emphasis on oncologic applications.

FLT

Deregulated cell cycle progression is a hallmark of cancer.[10] Accordingly, most therapeutic drugs have been designed to inhibit cell proliferation

[a] Department of Nuclear Medicine, King Hussein Medical Center, PO Box 855028, Amman 11855, Jordan
[b] Department of Nuclear Medicine, Technische Universität München, Ismaninger Strasse 22, Munich 81675, Germany
* Corresponding author.
E-mail address: ken.herrmann@tum.de

PET Clin 5 (2010) 363–374
doi:10.1016/j.cpet.2010.04.002

and/or induce apoptosis. In vivo assessment of proliferation is therefore a promising tool for assessment of response to cancer treatments targeting proliferating cells. Imaging of proliferation potentially allows not only better differentiation between benign and malign processes but also noninvasive grading of tumor aggressiveness.[7,11–14]

Noninvasive assessment of tumor growth and DNA synthesis might be appropriate for assessing proliferative activity in malignant tumors. So far, several DNA precursors have been investigated including [11C]thymidine, which represents the native pyrimidine analog used for DNA synthesis in vivo.[6] Because of the short half-life of 11C and rapid degradation of [11C]thymidine, this tracer was considered less suitable for clinical use.

Recently, FLT (the thymidine analogue 3'-deoxy-3'-[18F]fluorothymidine) was suggested for noninvasive assessment of proliferation and more specific tumor imaging.[15] The effort to synthesize FLT is similar to that of the standard radiotracer FDG.[16] FLT, which is derived from the cytostatic drug azidovudine (AZT), has been reported to be stable in vitro and to accumulate in proliferating tissues and malignant tumors.[17] Thymidine kinase 1 was revealed as the key enzyme responsible for the intracellular trapping of FLT.[18,19] Recently, a significant correlation of tumor proliferation and FLT uptake in various malignant tumors has been described, including breast cancer,[20] colorectal cancer,[21] lung cancer,[22] gliomas,[23,24] and lymphomas.[25]

The rationale of investigating FLT-PET for imaging of sarcoma is that the accuracy of FDG-PET for tumor grading and differentiation between benign and malignant tumors can be reduced by nonspecific uptake in inflammatory cells and aggressive benign tumors.[6–8] Several investigators reported a significantly higher uptake of FDG in high-grade compared with low-grade sarcomas, whereas benign and grade 1 sarcomas could not be reliably differentiated.[7,11–14]

In a prospective study with a total of 22 patients, the authors have recently shown that the proliferation marker FLT was suitable for imaging malignant bone or soft tissue tumors with a sensitivity of 100% (17/17). Mean FLT-SUV in benign lesions was 0.7, and 1.3 in low-grade sarcoma; 4.1 and 6.1 in grade 2 and grade 3 tumors respectively. FLT but not FDG uptake correlated significantly with tumor grading ($r = 0.71$ vs $r = 0.01$), and a cutoff value of 2.0 for FLT-SUV discriminated between low- and high-grade tumors. The authors concluded that FLT is a suitable PET tracer for imaging malignant bone or soft tissue tumors (Fig. 1). Moreover, uptake of FLT, but not FDG, correlated significantly with the tumor grade, suggesting FLT is a superior PET tracer for noninvasive grading of sarcomas.[26]

In a further study, Cobben and colleagues[27] investigated FLT-PET in soft tissue sarcomas of the extremities in a series of 19 patients. This study revealed that FLT-PET detects primary tumors and local recurrence of soft tissue sarcoma with a high accuracy and can also distinguish between low-grade (grade 1) and high-grade (grade 2 and 3) tumors. SUVs and tumor to nontumor ratios showed a significant correlation with the mitotic index, the proliferation marker MIB-1 as well as with the French and Japanese grading systems ($r = 0.55–0.75$). Tumors were visualized with high contrast, revealing mean SUVs of 0.9 and 2.8 for low- and high-grade tumors, respectively. Mean tumor to nontumor ratios were 1.9 and 6.0 for low- and high-grade tumors, respectively. These results show that FLT-PET was able to differentiate between low- and high-grade soft tissue sarcoma according to the French grading system. However, no differentiation could be made between benign and low-grade malignant soft tissue tumors.

In daily clinical practice, differentiation between benign and malignant tumors is based on histologic analysis of biopsied lesions including mitotic index and immunostaining of proliferating cells (eg, using the Ki-67 specific antibody MIB-1). However, the prognostic value of the proliferation fraction as assessed by immunohistochemistry remains a matter of debate. A biopsy is required in all cases, but in high-grade sarcoma it is suggested that 1 lesion is representative of all sarcoma lesions. In patients with low-grade sarcoma, the heterogeneity of tumor proliferation frequently cannot be identified except when biopsies from several tumor manifestation sites are performed. Therefore, transformation to a more aggressive histology may be underestimated. In patients with low-grade sarcoma, whole-body FLT-PET may indicate progression in areas with increased FLT uptake and may guide biopsy for further verification.

There is considerable evidence that FLT-PET has the potential to visualize and measure the viability of tumor cells during or early after chemotherapy because it does not accumulate in inflammatory cells.[28] However, the role of FLT-PET in measuring the response of musculoskeletal tumors to treatment has been scarcely investigated.

Been and colleagues[29] studied the potential role of FLT-PET to measure response to hyperthermic isolated limb perfusion (HILP) in 10 patients with initially nonresectable soft tissue sarcoma of the

FLT-PET   FDG-PET/CT

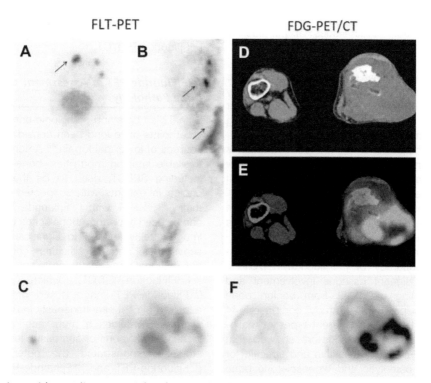

Fig. 1. A patient with a malignant peripheral nerve sheath tumor of the left distal femur reveals intense FLT uptake in the coronal (*A*), sagittal (*B*), and transaxial (*C*) FLT-PET scan displaying a significant increase of proliferation. Physiologic FLT uptake in the proliferating bone marrow of the sternum, ribs, and pelvis can be seen (*black arrows*). Corresponding FDG-PET/CT scan shows intense FDG uptake in projection of a soft tissue mass in the left distal femur; transaxial views of CT (*D*), fused PET/CT (*E*) and PET (*F*).

extremities. HILP with cytostatic agents has been introduced as a promising approach to render the most locally advanced soft tissue sarcomas resectable, thereby preventing the need for amputation. However, HILP with TNF-alpha and melphalan is an expensive treatment with possible serious side effects.[29,30] Moreover, conventional imaging techniques such as CT or MR imaging provide predominantly anatomic information such as tumor growth or tumor shrinkage, with limited information about tumor aggressiveness and biologic response to therapy. The results of this study revealed that high uptake of FLT-PET in soft tissue sarcomas showed a significant correlation with the mitotic index of the tumors (SUV$_{max}$: $r = 0.82$, $P = .004$; SUV$_{mean}$: $r = 0.87$, $P = .001$). Moreover, after HILP, the uptake of FLT decreased significantly ($P = .008$ and $P = .002$ for SUV$_{max}$ and SUV$_{mean}$, respectively). Tumors with initially high FLT uptake showed a better response to HILP ($r = 0.64$, $P<.05$). In this study, software fusion of PET images with images from conventional imaging modalities revealed the heterogeneity of the tumors before and after HILP.

[^{18}F]FLUORIDE

The spatial resolution of technetium 99mTc methylene diphosphonate (99mTc-MDP) skeletal scintigraphy and single photon emission-computed tomography (SPECT) affects their sensitivity for detection of musculoskeletal lesions. Thus, the transition to better resolution of PET or PET/CT contributes unique information about the metabolic activity of musculoskeletal lesions.[31] However, several researchers concluded that PET using FDG as tracer is not sensitive for osteoblastic lesions.[32,33]

[^{18}F]Fluoride is a bone-imaging agent that can be used for PET imaging. PET or PET/CT for detection of skeletal lesions seems to be feasible with the positron emitter ^{18}F offering a suitable half-life (110 min). After diffusing into the extracellular fluid of bone, the fluoride ion is exchanged for a hydroxyl group in the bone crystal and forms fluoroapatite, which then deposits at the bone surface where turnover is greatest.[34,35] Uptake of the fluoride ion (^{18}F) is 2-fold higher than that of 99mTc polyphosphonates. The combination of the better spatial resolution of PET and the improved image quality achieved by the favorable pharmacokinetic characteristics of [18F]fluoride has led to the use of [18F]fluoride-PET in the evaluation of skeletal lesions.

Increased uptake has been detected in sclerotic metastases and lytic lesions, with a statistically significant superiority of [18F]fluoride-PET over planar bone scintigraphy or SPECT in detecting benign and malignant bone pathology.[36–38]

[18F]Fluoride scans also show positive findings in nonmalignant bone lesions leading to a low specificity for differentiation between malignant and benign lesions. As in the case of bone scintigraphy, lesions detected on [18F]fluoride-PET often require correlation with other imaging modalities for further validation.[36]

Even-Sapir and colleagues[39] investigated the diagnostic accuracy of [18F]fluoride-PET/CT in assessing malignant osseous involvement and in differentiating malignant from benign bone lesions. This prospective study comprised 44 oncologic patients with different types of malignant primaries. The investigators showed that [18F]fluoride-PET/CT is sensitive and specific for detection of osteolytic and osteosclerotic bone lesions. The sensitivity of PET/CT was superior to PET alone in differentiating malignant from benign bone lesions in lesion- and patient-based analyses. PET/CT accurately differentiated malignant from benign bone lesions and possibly assisted in identifying a potential reason for the presence of bone pain in oncologic patients. For most lesions, the anatomic data provided by the low-dose CT of the PET/CT study obviate the need to perform an additional full-dose diagnostic CT for correlation purposes.

99mTc-MDP bone scintigraphy, FDG-PET, and [18F]fluoride-PET are different functional imaging approaches for assessment of malignant bone involvement. Because the 3 radiopharmaceuticals differ in their pharmacokinetic characteristics, they also differ in sensitivity in the detection of bone lesions in many malignant diseases. Moreover, the population investigated has a major effect on the results of studies assessing the performance of each approach.[35,40–46] Iagaru and colleagues[47] demonstrated in a prospective pilot study comprising 14 patients (6 patients with musculoskeletal tumors) the feasibility of combined [18F]fluoride/FDG administration followed by a single PET/CT scan for cancer detection. This combined method opens the possibility for improved patient care and reduction in health care costs.

Large prospective studies comparing [18F]fluoride-PET/CT with bone scintigraphy or FDG-PET including cost-effectiveness analysis are mandatory to identify clinical situations or patient populations that warrant the replacement of the more commonly used imaging studies by [18F]fluoride-PET/CT.

[18F]Fluoride-PET in Assessment of Benign Bone Pathology

Spinal disorders and pathologic conditions of the facet joints have long been considered common sources of lower back pain.[48] Among the various available imaging modalities, bone scintigraphy, including SPECT, used to be the modality of choice in patients with suspected bone abnormality.[49–53] PET with [18F]fluoride as the tracer can be used to perform bone scans with improved image quality leading to significantly improved sensitivities and specificities compared with conventional bone scintigraphy and SPECT.[54]

[18F]Fluoride-PET/CT, which consists of [18F]fluoride-PET images fused with CT images acquired almost simultaneously in PET/CT hybrid scanners, provides a more accurate anatomic localization of bone or soft tissue lesions. Recent studies demonstrated the potential role of [18F]fluoride-PET and [18F]fluoride-PET/CT in the diagnosis and evaluation of bone abnormalities in adolescent and young patients with back pain.[55,56] Lim and colleagues[57] performed [18F]fluoride-PET in 94 young patients. Focal abnormalities were present in 52 out of 94 patients. Of the 52 patients, 34% had abnormalities suggestive of pars/pedicle stress, 16% of a spinous process, 14% of a vertebral body abnormality, and 3% of abnormality related to the sacroiliac joint. Ovadia and colleagues[56] performed [18F]fluoride-PET/CT scans on 15 adolescents (mean age 14 years) with severe back pain. The patients had undergone several imaging studies including radiography, and in some cases 99mTc-MDP bone scan including SPECT; however, all of these diagnostic studies failed to determine the origin of the back pain. In this study, 10 of 15 (67%) patients showed abnormal uptake in the [18F]fluoride-PET/CT and were found to have bone abnormalities that included osteoid osteoma (2 patients), spondylolysis (4 patients), and fractures (4 patients). The 5 patients with negative [18F]fluoride-PET/CT studies had no bone pathology and recovered spontaneously.

Gamilie and El-Maghraby[58] reported their experience in the assessment of back pain in 67 adult patients using [18F]fluoride-PET/CT and suspected facetogenic pain; 25 individuals of this group had previous operative procedures of the spine. The investigators reported that in 42 patients with back pain and no previous operative procedures, [18F]fluoride-PET/CT showed a high sensitivity (88%; 37/42) in identifying the origin for the bone pain. In 25 patients with prior lumbar fusion or laminectomy, PET/CT showed positive uptake in 76% of the patients (19/25). [18F]Fluoride-PET/CT showed uptake in all patients (100%) with a history of pain after lumbar fusion, whereas in the laminectomy subgroup, only 11 patients (65%) showed positive focal uptake. The investigators concluded that there is a potential role for [18F]fluoride-PET/CT in the assessment of adult patients with back pain. However, it is preferable to use PET in situations when pathology cannot be identified by CT and/or MR imaging; moreover, [18F]fluoride-PET/CT might have a promising role in identifying underlying reasons of persistent back pain following surgical interventions on vertebrae.

RADIOLABELED AMINO ACID TRACERS

Radiolabeled amino acids have proved to be useful for imaging in several clinical scenarios.[59–62] The tumor uptake is thought to reflect increased amino acid metabolism in cancer cells, such as increased active transport and protein synthesis.

Kole and colleagues[63] investigated the relationship of PET using FDG or amino acids tracer L-[1-11C]tyrosine (TYR) with histopathologic findings in soft tissue tumors, before and after therapy. This study included 55 patients. In 28 patients, a second PET study was performed after therapy. Histopathologic parameters included tumor grade, mitotic rate, proliferative activity, and estimation of the amount of necrosis. Results of this study showed correlation between metabolic rate of glucose consumption, tumor grade, and mitotic rate but not with proliferation or necrosis. After therapy, no correlation with mitotic rate was observed. On the other hand, protein synthesis rate correlated with tumor grade, mitotic rate, and proliferation. After therapy, correlation with mitosis and proliferation had improved, and a negative correlation was found between protein synthesis rate and the extent of necrosis. This study demonstrates a clear correlation between FDG-PET and TYR-PET on the one hand and several histopathologic tumor parameters on the other. This correlation exists even though the tumor metabolic activity was compared with histopathologic parameters from a biopsy specimen that may not be representative of the whole tumor. The investigators concluded that FDG and TYR are efficient to give an in vivo indication of histologic tumor parameters. However, FDG gives a better indication of tumor grade, whereas TYR is more accurate in predicting mitotic rate and proliferation, especially after therapy.

Although amino acids labeled with carbon 11 are suitable for PET imaging, the short half-life of 11C (20 minutes) limits availability of these tracers to PET centers with an in-house cyclotron, preventing their widespread use. Moreover, new tracers such as amino acids labeled with fluorine 18, [18F]fluoroethyl-L-tyrosine (FET) or L-[3-18F]-α-methyltyrosine (FMT), have been introduced as more suitable radiopharmaceuticals for PET imaging.[64–66] These tracers have the advantages of a longer half-life ($t_{1/2} = 110$ minutes) and a simple and efficient synthesis. The physical properties of these tracers are suitable for the acquisition of whole-body PET scans, and they are promising for use in clinical oncology.

Tomiyoshi and colleagues[65] developed FMT as a tumor-detecting amino acid tracer for PET imaging. In contrast to radiolabeled methionine and tyrosine, FMT, an amino acid analogue, is accumulated in tumor cells solely via an amino acid transport system.[64] This process is unique to FMT; by contrast, FDG is used in glucose metabolism and metabolically trapped in the cells.[67] Watanabe and colleagues[68] evaluated the potential of FMT-PET to distinguish malignant tumors and benign mass forming lesions in the musculoskeletal system, compared with FDG-PET. This prospective study comprised 75 patients and the results were analyzed in 3 categories. First, for detection of musculoskeletal tumors, FMT and FDG were equally useful agents for the detection of bone and soft tissue tumors. FMT-PET visualized all malignancies and a similar percentage of benign lesions as detected by FDG-PET. Second, for differentiation of benign lesions and malignant tumors, FDG seems to be unsuitable for discriminating benign lesions from sarcomas with relatively low malignancy. Besides, with a cutoff value of 1.2 for FMT-SUV_{mean}, the sensitivity and specificity of FMT-PET for differentiation of benign and malignant musculoskeletal lesions were 72.7% and 84.9%, respectively, resulting in an overall accuracy of 81.3% which was clearly higher than that of FDG-PET. In particular, 13 out of 18 benign lesions that were false-positive on FDG-PET were evaluated correctly into the low-SUV_{mean} group on FMT-PET. Third, for grading malignancy, a significant correlation was found between malignant tumor grade and SUV in FMT- and FDG-PET ($P = .656$ and 0.815, respectively), despite the inclusion of malignancies originating from many different types of tissue. The investigators concluded that FMT may be superior to FDG for differentiation of benign and malignant tumors, and thus be important for preoperative planning. However, in a recent report by Ghigi and colleagues,[69] FMT was less accurate than FDG in discrimination between complete responders and partial responders regarding neoadjuvant chemoradiotherapy for soft tissue sarcomas. It is clear that further prospective studies including a larger number of patients are necessary to validate these preliminary applications.

FET is a radiolabeled analog of tyrosine that is not metabolized and not incorporated into proteins but is actively transported into tumor cells, and is sufficient for satellite distribution. In accordance with findings obtained with other radiolabeled amino acids,[70,71] first clinical experience with FMT suggests that it is not significantly incorporated into inflammatory cells.[72] Assuming a similar effect for FET, a more tumor-specific uptake can be expected in contrast to FDG, which shows not only accumulation in cancer cells but also in inflammatory cells.[73,74] Kaim and colleagues[75] suggested in a preliminary report that FET-PET is more suitable than FDG-PET for differentiating infection and recurrent tumor, because the immunologic host response will not be labeled and inflammation can be excluded. Nevertheless, still further clinical studies are required to prove that tumor detection with FET is at least as sensitive as with FDG.

[18F]GALACTO-RGD

The integrin $\alpha v\beta 3$ is an interesting target for specific therapies in oncology, as it is highly expressed on activated endothelial cells during angiogenesis and plays an important role in the regulation of tumor growth, local invasiveness, and metastatic potential.[76,77] Potential therapeutic strategies include the use of humanized antibodies directed against $\alpha v\beta 3$ or cyclic pentapeptides with specific binding to $\alpha v\beta 3$.[78,79] A well-known disadvantage is that, in many cases, the expression of highly specific targets is limited to a subset of patients depending on tumor type and stage. Hence, a strategy to non-invasively assess the intensity of $\alpha v\beta 3$ expression in humans would be of paramount importance for the selection of those patients most amenable to $\alpha v\beta 3$-targeted therapies.

Haubner and colleagues[80] developed the tracer [18F]galacto-RGD for PET of $\alpha v\beta 3$ expression. [18F]Galacto-RGD showed high affinity and selectivity for the $\alpha v\beta 3$ integrin in vitro, receptor-specific accumulation in a murine $\alpha v\beta 3$-positive osteosarcoma tumor model, and high metabolic stability and predominantly renal elimination. Moreover, the investigators demonstrated in two other reports that this tracer can be successfully used to image $\alpha v\beta 3$-positive tumors in patients with cancer, with good image quality and a favorable biodistribution.[81,82]

Beer and colleagues[83] showed in a prospective study comprising 19 patients (10 with musculoskeletal tumors) that PET using [18F]galacto-RGD can correctly identify the level of $\alpha v\beta 3$ expression in man, therefore, this facilitates the noninvasive assessment of angiogenesis and the metastatic potential of tumors by molecular imaging with PET. The results of this study demonstrated that well-differentiated tumors, such as low-grade liposarcomas, showed low or no $\alpha v\beta 3$ expression in immunohistochemistry and no substantial uptake of [18F]galacto-RGD, whereas high-grade sarcomas showed higher tracer uptake, a higher microvessel density of $\alpha v\beta 3$-positive vessels and $\alpha v\beta 3$-positive tumor cells. There was no correlation between tumor size and [18F]galacto-RGD uptake, which shows that a higher tracer uptake was not simply caused by a larger tumor volume. However, the diversity of uptake intensity suggests that the intensity of $\alpha v\beta 3$ expression depends on various factors and is not uniformly high in all tumor entities at all times (**Fig. 2**). The higher degree of $\alpha v\beta 3$ expression on tumor cells in more aggressive tumors can be explained by the important role of $\alpha v\beta 3$ in cell migration, invasion, and metastatic activity.[84–87]

Potential future applications for PET using [18F]galacto-RGD are various. In inflammatory processes, for example, it might be used to assess disease activity. It might also be applied for monitoring angiogenesis during antiangiogenic therapies. In this respect, PET might have some advantages compared with dynamic contrast-enhanced MR imaging, which is, up to now, the modality most commonly applied in clinical studies. Dynamic contrast-enhanced MR imaging data need to be analyzed using kinetic modeling techniques and are difficult to interpret because dynamic contrast-enhanced MR imaging represents a complex summation of vascular permeability, blood flow, vascular surface area, and interstitial pressure.[88] The approach of targeting the integrin $\alpha v\beta 3$ on the other hand is very specific. Moreover, only a limited part of the body can be examined with dynamic contrast-enhanced MR imaging, whereas with PET, functional imaging of the entire body can be provided. However, this ultimate value of PET imaging of $\alpha v\beta 3$ expression still has to be proved in future correlative prospective studies. It might well be that functional imaging and molecular imaging of angiogenesis provide complementary information on tumor biology. In this respect, great promise lies in combined MR-PET imaging, which allows for a one-stop-shop approach for imaging of

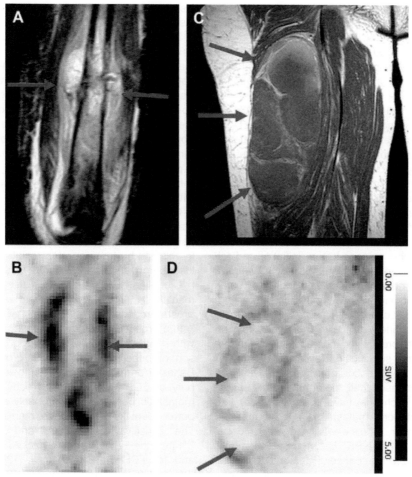

Fig. 2. Two patients with sarcomas of the thigh (*arrows*). Left: a patient with osteosarcoma of the right femur (*A, B*), Right: a patient with a liposarcoma (*C, D*). In the MR image (*A, C*: T1 weighted contrast enhanced; coronal) large tumors with intense contrast enhancement can be seen. The corresponding [^{18}F]Galacto-RGD PET (*B, D,* coronal slices) shows different uptake patterns in both patients: in the osteosarcoma, intense tracer uptake can be seen predominantly in the tumor periphery, whereas in the liposarcoma there is mostly faint tracer uptake, with some focal areas of more intense tracer uptake, suggesting heterogeneous avb3 expression in these 2 tumors.

morphologic, functional, and molecular parameters of musculoskeletal disease.[89]

CHOLINE

Choline is an essential component of the cell membrane that is presumably taken up via a choline-specific transporter protein.[90] In malignant cells choline kinase, which catalyzes the phosphorylation of choline, is up-regulated. In 1998 Hara and colleagues[91] introduced choline labeled with carbon 11 for imaging. [^{11}C]Choline uptake is significantly higher in malignant tumors than in benign tumors and correlates well with the degree of FDG accumulation of the lesion.[92] Moreover, compared with FDG, the physiologic

background level in the urinary tract is low, which may be a result of incomplete tubular reabsorption of the intact tracer, or enhanced excretion of labeled oxidative metabolites like betaine.[90,93,94] [^{11}C]Choline uptake is physiologic in the liver, pancreas, kidney, and duodenum. In a nonfasting state [^{11}C]choline is also secreted into phospholipid-rich pancreatic juice.[92]

Tateishi and colleagues[92] investigated the potential role of [^{11}C]choline-PET for staging of bone and soft tissue sarcomas. In a retrospective study comprising 16 patients they compared it with conventional diagnostic tools including MR imaging, CT, and bone scintigraphy. Using [^{11}C]choline-PET/CT, the M stage was correctly assigned in 15 patients (94%), whereas the accuracy of conventional imaging in the M stage was 81% (P = .617). TNM stage was correctly assessed in 15 of 16 patients (94%) with [^{11}C]choline-PET/CT but only in 8 of 16 patients with conventional imaging (50%, P = .023). Eight patients were understaged by conventional imaging (missing skip metastases of soft tissues n = 2 and small nodal metastases n = 6). The investigators concluded that [^{11}C]choline-PET/CT plays an important role for staging in patients with bone and soft tissue sarcomas, increasing the accuracy of overall TNM-staging compared with conventional imaging.

Early detection of metastatic bone disease and the definition of its extent and aggressiveness are crucial for proper staging and restaging in prostate cancer; it is particularly important in high-risk primary disease before initiating radical prostatectomy or radiation therapy. Different patterns of bone metastases, such as early marrow-based involvement, sclerotic, lytic, and mixed changes can be seen. Bone scintigraphy has been routinely used in the evaluation of patients with prostate cancer, but has limited sensitivity and specificity. Several PET tracers based either on detection of increased glycolysis (FDG) or increased cell membrane proliferation ([^{11}C] and [^{18}F]choline) have been tested for the evaluation of bone metastases in patients with prostate cancer. Choline was suggested to be superior to FDG as a PET tracer in detection and staging of prostate cancer.[4,95] Recently, [^{11}C] and [^{18}F] labeled choline PET have shown promising results in the evaluation of patients with prostate cancer.[95–97] [^{11}C]Choline has the limitation of availability because of its short half-life.[91] Recent successful labeling of choline compounds with ^{18}F overcomes some of the limitations of ^{11}C, such as the short half-life, and provides more flexibility for imaging protocols and availability.[98]

In a recent report, Beheshti and colleagues[98] evaluated the potential role of [^{18}F]choline-PET/CT (FCH-PET/CT) for the assessment of bone metastases in patients with prostate cancer. Furthermore, they assessed the pattern of metabolic uptake of FCH in relation to morphologic changes seen on CT. Seventy patients were included in this prospective study. Results revealed that the sensitivity, specificity, and accuracy of FCH-PET/CT in detecting bone metastases were 79%, 97%, and 84%, respectively. Lesion-based analysis showed 262 lesions with increased uptake on FCH-PET, of which 210 lesions were interpreted as bone metastases. No detectable morphological changes were found in 49 (24%) lesions on CT, which can be most likely explained by bone marrow metastases. The mean SUV$_{max}$ in all malignant lesions was 8.1 ± 3.9. Furthermore, lytic metastases showed a higher FCH uptake (mean SUV 11 ± 3.2) compared with sclerotic metastases (mean 7.6 ± 3.0). A Hounsfield unit (HU) level greater than 825 was associated with an absence of FCH uptake. Almost all of the FCH-negative sclerotic lesions were detected in patients who were under hormone therapy, which raises the possibility that these lesions might no longer be viable. It is obvious from these results that FCH-PET/CT plays a promising role in the early detection of bone metastases in patients with prostate cancer.

In a previously published prospective study with 45 patients the additional impact of [^{11}C]choline-PET/CT in the assessment of skeletal metastases in staging and restaging of patients with prostate cancer was also shown.[99] In this study, low-dose CT results in improved localization and lesion characterization. Overall, [^{11}C]choline-PET/CT changed disease management in 11 (24%) of 45 patients with advanced prostate cancer.

In a prospective study comparing FCH-PET/CT with [^{18}F]fluoride-PET/CT scanning for the detection of bone metastases from prostate cancer, Beheshti and colleagues[100] suggested a superiority of FCH-PET/CT for the early detection of metastatic bone disease probably as a result of better identification of bone marrow infiltration. The sensitivity, specificity, and accuracy of [^{18}F]fluoride-PET/CT was 81%, 93%, and 86% and for FCH was 74% (P = .12), 99% (P = .01) and 85%, respectively. FCH-PET/CT led to a change in disease management in 2 out of 38 patients as a result of the early detection of bone marrow metastases. [^{18}F]Fluoride-PET/CT identified more lesions in some patients compared with FCH-PET/CT but did not change patient management. This study also clarified that both agents were more sensitive for lytic lesions than sclerotic lesions. Moreover, a correlation was found between SUVs and the density of the sclerotic bone lesions. However, in patients with FCH-negative suspicious sclerotic lesions, a second bone-seeking agent like [^{18}F]fluoride may be useful.

The high accuracy of [^{11}C]choline-PET/CT was also confirmed in 2 recently published reports comparing [^{11}C]choline-PET/CT with whole-body MR and diffusion-weighted MR for assessment of bone metastases in patients with prostate cancer.[101,102] In summary, [^{11}C]choline-PET/CT provides important additional information regarding the staging and restaging of bone metastases in patients with prostate cancer and in patients with soft tissue sarcomas. In the future, combination of PET information provided by

[^{11}C]choline and diffusion-weighted MR seems promising especially in consideration of combined MR-PET scanners.

REFERENCES

1. Landis SH, Murray T, Bolden S, et al. Cancer statistics, 1999. CA Cancer J Clin 1999;49:8–31.
2. Erlemann R, Reiser MF, Peters PE, et al. Musculoskeletal neoplasms: static and dynamic Gd-DTPA-enhanced MR imaging. Radiology 1989;171:767–73.
3. Verstraete KL, VanderWoude HJ, Hogendoorn, et al. Dynamic contrast-enhanced MR imaging of musculoskeletal tumors: basic principles and clinical applications. J Magn Reson Imaging 1996;5:311–21.
4. von Schulthess GK, Steinert HC, HanyTF, et al. Integrated PET/CT: current applications and future directions. Radiology 2006;238:405–22.
5. Bastiaannet E, Groen H, Jager PL, et al. The value of FDG-PET in the detection, grading and response to therapy of soft tissue and bone sarcomas; a systematic review and meta-analysis. Cancer Treat Rev 2004;30:83–101.
6. Aoki J, Watanabe H, Shinozaki T, et al. FDG PET of primary benign and malignant bone tumors: standardized uptake value in 52 lesions. Radiology 2001;219:774–7.
7. Kubota R, Kubota K, Yamada S, et al. Microautoradiographic study for the differentiation of intratumoral macrophages, granulation tissues and cancer cells by the dynamics of fluorine-18-fluorodeoxyglucose uptake. J Nucl Med 1994;35:104–12.
8. Shreve PD, Anzai Y, Wahl RL. Pitfalls in oncologic diagnosis with FDG PET imaging: physiologic and benign variants. Radiographics 1999;19:61–77.
9. Nieweg OE, Pruim J, van Ginkel RJ, et al. Fluorine-18-fluorodeoxyglucose PET imaging of soft-tissue sarcoma. J Nucl Med 1996;37:257–61.
10. Hanahan D, Weinberg RA. The hallmarks of cancer. Cell 2000;100(1):57–70.
11. Adler LP, Blair HF, Markley JT, et al. Noninvasive grading of musculoskeletal tumors using PET. J Nucl Med 1991;32:1508–12.
12. Eary JF, Conrad EU, Bruckner JD, et al. Quantitative [F-18]fluorodeoxyglucose positron emission tomography in pretreatment and grading of sarcoma. Clin Cancer Res 1998;4:1215–20.
13. Schulte M, Brecht-Krauss D, Heymer B, et al. Fluorodeoxyglucose positron emission tomography of soft tissue tumours: is a non-invasive determination of biological activity possible? Eur J Nucl Med 1999;26:599–605.
14. Schulte M, Brecht-Kraus D, Heymer B, et al. Grading of tumors and tumorlike lesions of

bone: evaluation by FDG-PET. J Nucl Med 2000;41:1695–701.
15. Shields AF, Grierson JR, Dohmen BM, et al. Imaging proliferation in vivo with [F-18]FLT and positron emission tomography. Nat Med 1998; 4(11):1334–6.
16. Machulla HJ, Blocher A, Kuntzsch M, et al. Simplified labeling approach for synthesizing 3′-deoxy-3′-[^{18}F]fluorothymidine ([^{18}F]FLT). J Radioanal Nucl Chem 2000;243(3):843–6.
17. Wells P, Gunn RN, Alison M, et al. Assessment of proliferation in vivo using 2-[(11)C]thymidine positron emission tomography in advanced intraabdominal malignancies. Cancer Res 2002; 62(20):5698–702.
18. Rasey JS, Grierson JR, Wiens LW, et al. Validation of FLT uptake as a measure of thymidine kinase-1 activity in A549 carcinoma cells. J Nucl Med 2002;43(9):1210–7.
19. Barthel H, Perumal M, Latigo J, et al. The uptake of 3′-deoxy-3′-[^{18}F]fluorothymidine into L5178Y tumours in vivo is dependent on thymidine kinase 1 protein levels. Eur J Nucl Med Mol Imaging 2005;32(3):257–63.
20. Kenny LM, Vigushin DM, Al-Nahhas A, et al. Quantification of cellular proliferation in tumor and normal tissues of patients with breast cancer by [^{18}F]fluorothymidine-positron emission tomography imaging: evaluation of analytical methods. Cancer Res 2005;65(21):10104–12.
21. Francis DL, Visvikis D, Costa DC, et al. Potential impact of [^{18}F]3′-deoxy-3′-fluorothymidine versus [^{18}F]fluoro-2-deoxy-D-glucose in positron emission tomography for colorectal cancer. Eur J Nucl Med Mol Imaging 2003;30(7):988–94.
22. Buck AK, Schirrmeister H, Hetzel M, et al. 3-Deoxy-3-[(18)F]fluorothymidine-positron emission tomography for noninvasive assessment of proliferation in pulmonary nodules. Cancer Res 2002;62(12): 3331–4.
23. Chen W, Cloughesy T, Kamdar N, et al. Imaging proliferation in brain tumors with ^{18}F-FLT PET: comparison with ^{18}F-FDG. J Nucl Med 2005; 46(6):945–52.
24. Choi SJ, Kim JS, Kim JH, et al. [^{18}F]3′-deoxy-3′-fluorothymidine PET for the diagnosis and grading of brain tumors. Eur J Nucl Med Mol Imaging 2005; 32(6):653–9.
25. Wagner M, Seitz U, Buck A, et al. 3′-[^{18}F]fluoro-3′-deoxythymidine ([^{18}F]-FLT) as positron emission tomography tracer for imaging proliferation in a murine B-cell lymphoma model and in the human disease. Cancer Res 2003;63(10):2681–7.
26. Buck AK, Herrmann K, Buschenfelde CZ, et al. Imaging bone and soft tissue tumors with the proliferation marker [^{18}F]fluorodeoxythymidine. Clin Cancer Res 2008;14(10):2970–7.

27. Cobben DC, Elsinga PH, Suurmeijer AJ, et al. Detection and grading of soft tissue sarcomas of the extremities with ^{18}F-3-fluoro-3-deoxy-L-thymidine. Clin Cancer Res 2004;10:1685–90.

28. van Waarde A, Cobben DC, Suurmeijer AJ, et al. Selectivity of ^{18}F-FLT and ^{18}F-FDG for differentiating tumor from inflammation in a rodent model. J Nucl Med 2004;45:695–700.

29. Been LB, Suurmeijer AJH, Elsinga PH, et al. ^{18}F-Fluorodeoxythymidine PET for evaluating the response to hyperthermic isolated limb perfusion for locally advanced soft-tissue sarcomas. J Nucl Med 2007;48:367–72.

30. Zwaveling JH, Maring JK, Mulder AB, et al. Effects of hyperthermic isolated limb perfusion with recombinant tumor necrosis factor alpha and melphalan on the human fibrinolytic system. Cancer Res 1996;56:3948–53.

31. Feldman F, van Heertum R, Manos C. [18]FDG PET scanning of benign and malignant musculoskeletal lesions. Skeletal Radiol 2003;32:201–8.

32. Uematsu T, Yuen S, Yukisawa S, et al. Comparison of FDG PET and SPECT for detection of bone metastases in breast cancer. AJR Am J Roentgenol 2005;184:1266–73.

33. Nakai T, Okuyama C, Kubota T, et al. Pitfalls of FDG-PET for the diagnosis of osteoblastic bone metastases in patients with breast cancer. Eur J Nucl Med Mol Imaging 2005;32:1253–8.

34. Schiepers C, Nuytes J, Bormans G, et al. Fluoride kinetics of the axial skeleton measured in vivo with fluorine-18-fluoride PET. J Nucl Med 1997;38:1970–6.

35. Cook JR, Fogelman I. The role of positron emission tomography in the management of bone metastases. Cancer 2000;88:2927–33.

36. Schirrmeister H, Guhlmann A, Elsner K, et al. Sensitivity in detecting osseous lesions depends on anatomic localization: planar bone scintigraphy versus ^{18}F PET. J Nucl Med 1999;40:1623–9.

37. Schirrmeister H, Guhlnamm A, Kotzerke J, et al. Early detection and accurate description of extent of metastatic bone disease in breast cancer with fluoride ion and positron emission tomography. J Clin Oncol 1999;17:2381–9.

38. Hoegerle S, Juengling F, Otte A, et al. Combined FDG and F-18-fluoride whole body PET: a feasible two-in-one approach to cancer imaging. Radiology 1998;209:253–8.

39. Even-Sapir E, Metser U, Flusser G. Assessment of malignant skeletal disease: initial experience with ^{18}F-fluoride PET/CT and comparison between ^{18}F-fluoride PET and ^{18}F-fluoride PET/CT. J Nucl Med 2004;45:272–8.

40. Bury T, Barreto A, Daenen F, et al. Flourine-18 deoxyglucose positron emission tomography for the detection of bone metastases in patients with non-small cell lung cancer. Eur J Nucl Med 1998;25:1244–7.

41. Moog F, Kotzerke J, Reske SN. FDG PET can replace bone scintigraphy in primary staging of malignant lymphoma. J Nucl Med 1999;40:1407–13.

42. Marom EM, McAdams P, Erasmus JJ, et al. Staging non-small cell lung cancer with whole-body PET. Radiology 1999;212:803–9.

43. Franzius F, Sciuk J, Daldrup-Link HE, et al. FDG-PET for detection of osseous metastases from malignant primary bone tumours: comparison with bone scintigraphy. Eur J Nucl Med 2000;27:1305–11.

44. Daldrup-Link HE, Franzius C, Link TM, et al. Whole body MR imaging for detection of bone metastases in children and young adults. AJR Am J Roentgenol 2001;177:229–36.

45. Cook GJ, Houston S, Rubens R, et al. Detection of bone metastases in breast cancer by [18]FDG PET: differing metabolic activity in osteoblastic and osteolytic lesions. J Clin Oncol 1998;16:3375–9.

46. Shreve PD, Grossman HB, Gross MD, et al. Metastatic prostate cancer: initial finding of PT 2-deoxyglucose-[F-18]fluoro-D-glucose. Radiology 1996;199:751–6.

47. Iagaru A, Mittra E, Yaghoubi S, et al. Novel strategy for a cocktail ^{18}F-fluoride and ^{18}F-FDG PET/CT scan for evaluation of malignancy: results of the pilot-phase study. J Nucl Med 2009;50:501–5.

48. Pneumaticos SG, Chatziioannou SN, Hipp JA, et al. Low back pain: prediction of short-term outcome of facet joint injection with bone scintigraphy. Radiology 2006;238:693–8.

49. Ryan RJ, Gibson T, Fogelman I. The identification of spinal pathology in chronic low back pain using single photon emission computed tomography. Nucl Med Commun 1992;13:497–502.

50. Holder LE, Machin JL, Asdourian PL, et al. Planar and high-resolution SPECT bone imaging in the diagnosis of facet syndrome. J Nucl Med 1995;36:37–44.

51. Dolan AL, Ryan PJ, Arden NK, et al. The value of SPECT scans in identifying back pain likely to benefit from facet joint injection. Br J Rheumatol 1996;35:1269–73.

52. Lusins JO, Cicoria AD, Goldsmith SJ. SPECT and lumbar MRI in back pain with emphasis on changes in end plates in association with disc degeneration. J Neuroimaging 1998;8:78–82.

53. De Maeseneer M, Lenchik L, Everaert H, et al. Evaluation of lower back pain with bone scintigraphy and SPECT. Radiographics 1999;19:901–12 [discussion: 912–4].

54. Bridges RL, Wiley CR, Christian JC, et al. An introduction to Na(18)F bone scintigraphy: basic principles, advanced imaging concepts, and case

examples. J Nucl Med Technol 2007;35:64–76 [quiz: 78–9].

55. Houseni M, Chamroonrat W, Zhuang H, et al. Facet joint arthropathy demonstrated on FDG-PET. Clin Nucl Med 2006;31:418–9.

56. Ovadia D, Metser U, Lievshitz G, et al. Back pain in adolescents: assessment with integrated ^{18}F-fluoride positron-emission tomography-computed tomography. J Pediatr Orthop 2007;27:90–3.

57. Lim R, Fahey FH, Drubach LA, et al. Early experience with fluorine-18 sodium fluoride bone PET in young patients with back pain. J Pediatr Orthop 2007;27:277–82.

58. Gamie S, El-Maghraby T. The role of PET/CT in evaluation of facet and disc abnormalities in patients with low back pain using ^{18}F-fluoride. Nucl Med Rev Cent East Eur 2008;11(1):17–21.

59. Langen KJ, Ziemons K, Kiwit JC, et al. 3-[^{123}I]iodo-alphamethyltyrosine and [methyl-^{11}C]-L-methionine uptake in cerebral gliomas: a comparative study using SPECT and PET. J Nucl Med 1997; 38:517–22.

60. Leskinen Kallio S, Ruotsalainen U, Nagren K, et al. Uptake of carbon-11-methionine and fluorodeoxyglucose in non-Hodgkin's lymphoma: a PET study. J Nucl Med 1991;32:1211–8.

61. Nettelbladt OS, Sundin AE, Valind SO, et al. Combined fluorine-18-FDG and carbon-11-methionine PET for diagnosis of tumors in lung and mediastinum. J Nucl Med 1998;39:640–7.

62. Leskinen Kallio S, Nagren K, Lehikoinen P, et al. Uptake of ^{11}C-methionine in breast cancer studied by PET. An association with the size of S-phase fraction. Br J Cancer 1991;64:1121–4.

63. Kole AC, Plaat BG, Hoekstra H, et al. FDG and L-[l-nC] tyrosine imaging of soft- tissue tumors before and after therapy. J Nucl Med 1999;40: 381–6.

64. Weber WA, Wester HJ, Grosu AL, et al. O-(2-[^{18}F]Fluoroethyl)-L-tyrosine and L-[methyl-^{11}C]methionine uptake in brain tumours: initial results of a comparative study. Eur J Nucl Med 2000;27: 542–9.

65. Tomiyoshi K, Amed K, Muhammad S, et al. Synthesis of isomers of ^{18}F-labelled amino acid radiopharmaceutical: position 2- and 3-L-^{18}F-alpha-methyltyrosine using a separation and purification system. Nucl Med Commun 1997;18:169–75.

66. Inoue T, Tomiyoshi K, Higuchi T, et al. Biodistribution studies on L-3-[fluorine-18]fluoro-alpha-methyl tyrosine: a potential tumor-detecting agent. J Nucl Med 1998;39:663–7.

67. Gallagher BM, Fowler JS, Gutterson NI, et al. Metabolic trapping as a principle of radiopharmaceutical design: some factors responsible for the biodistribution of [^{18}F] 2-deoxy-2-fluoro-D-glucose. J Nucl Med 1978;19:1154–61.

68. Watanabe H, Inoue T, Shinozaki T, et al. PET imaging of musculoskeletal tumours with fluorine-18α-methyltyrosine: comparison with fluorine-18 fluorodeoxyglucose PET. Eur J Nucl Med 2000;27: 1509–17.

69. Ghigi G, Micera R, Margherita A, et al. ^{11}C-Methionine vs. ^{18}F-FDG PET in soft tissue sarcoma patients treated with neoadjuvant therapy: preliminary results. In vivo 2009;23:105–10.

70. Kubota R, Kubota K, Yamada S, et al. Methionine uptake by tumor tissue: a microautoradiographic comparison with FDG. J Nucl Med 1995;36: 484–92.

71. Kubota K, Ishiwata K, Kubota R, et al. Feasibility of fluorine-18-fluorophenylalanine for tumor imaging compared with carbon-11-L-methionine. J Nucl Med 1996;7:320–32.

72. Inoue T, Koyama K, Oriuchi N, et al. Detection of malignant tumors: whole-body PET with fluorine 18 alpha-methyl tyrosine versus FDG-preliminary study. Radiology 2001;220:54–62.

73. Kubota K, Kubota R, Yamada S, et al. FDG accumulation in tumor tissue. J Nucl Med 1993;34: 419–21.

74. Kubota R, Yamada S, Kubota K, et al. Intratumoral distribution of fluorine-18-fluorodeoxyglucose in vivo: high accumulation in macrophages and granulation tissues studied by microautoradiography. J Nucl Med 1992;33:1972–80.

75. Kaim AH, Weber B, Kurrer MO, et al. ^{18}F-FDG and ^{18}F-FET uptake in experimental soft tissue infection. Eur J Nucl Med 2002;29:648–54.

76. Hood JD, Cheresh DA. Role of integrins in cell invasion and migration. Nat Rev Cancer 2002;2: 91–100.

77. Ruoslahti E. Specialization of tumor vasculature. Nat Rev Cancer 2002;2:83–90.

78. Dechantsreiter MA, Planker E, Matha B, et al. N-methylated cyclic RGD peptides as highly active and selective αvβ3 antagonists. J Med Chem 1999;42:3033–40.

79. Patel SR, Jenkins J, Papadopolous N, et al. Pilot study of vitaxinKan angiogenesis inhibitorKin patients with advanced leiomyosarcomas. Cancer 2001;92:1347–8.

80. Haubner R, Wester HJ, Weber WA, et al. Noninvasive imaging of αvβ3 integrin expression using ^{18}F-labeled RGD-containing glycopeptide and positron emission tomography. Cancer Res 2001; 61:1781–5.

81. Haubner R, Weber WA, Beer AJ, et al. Non-invasive visualization of the activated αvβ3 integrin in cancer patients by positron emission tomography and [^{18}F]galacto-RGD. PLoS Med 2005;2:e70.

82. Beer AJ, Haubner R, Goebel M, et al. Biodistribution and pharmacokinetics of the αvβ3 selective

tracer ^{18}F galacto-RGD in cancer patients. J Nucl Med 2005;46:1333–41.

83. Beer AJ, Haubner R, Sarbia M, et al. Positron emission tomography using [^{18}F]Galacto-RGD identifies the level of integrin $\alpha v \beta 3$ expression in man. Clin Cancer Res 2006;12(13):3942–9.

84. Felding-Habermann B. Integrin adhesion receptors in tumor metastasis. Clin Exp Metastasis 2003;20: 203–13.

85. Felding-Habermann B, O'Toole TE, Smith JW, et al. Integrin activation controls metastasis in human breast cancer. Proc Natl Acad Sci U S A 2001;98:1853–8.

86. Byzova TV, Kim W, Midura RJ, et al. Activation of integrin $\alpha v \beta 3$ regulates cell adhesion and migration to bone sialoprotein. Exp Cell Res 2000;254:299–308.

87. Stupack DG, Cheresh DA. A bit-role for integrins in apoptosis. Nat Cell Biol 2004;6:388–9.

88. McDonald DM, Choyke PL. Imaging of angiogenesis: from microscope to clinic. Nat Med 2003;9:713–25.

89. Judenhofer MS, Wehrl HF, Newport DF, et al. Simultaneous PET-MRI: a new approach for functional and morphological imaging. Nat Med 2008;14(4):459–65.

90. Ishidate K. Choline/ethanolamine kinase from mammalian tissues. Biochim Biophys Acta 1997; 1348:70–8.

91. Hara T, Kosaka N, Kishi H. PET imaging of prostate cancer using carbon-11-choline. J Nucl Med 1998; 39(6):990–5.

92. Tateishi U, Yamaguchi U, Maeda T, et al. Staging performance of carbon-11 choline positron emission tomography/computed tomography inpatients with bone and soft tissue sarcoma: comparison with conventional imaging. Cancer Sci 2006;97(10):1125–8.

93. Zhang H, Tian M, Oriuchi N, et al. ^{11}C-choline PET for the detection of bone and soft tissue tumours in comparison with FDG PET. Nucl Med Commun 2003;24:273–9.

94. Tian M, Zhang H, Oriuchi N, et al. Comparison of ^{11}C-choline PET and FDG PET for the differential diagnosis of malignant tumors. Eur J Nucl Med Mol Imaging 2004;31:1064–72.

95. Langsteger W, Heinisch M, Fogelman I. The role of fluorodeoxyglucose, ^{18}F-dihydroxyphenylalanine, ^{18}F-choline, and ^{18}F-fluoride in bone imaging with emphasis on prostate and breast. Semin Nucl Med 2006;36:73–92.

96. Cimitan M, Bortolus R, Morassut S, et al. [^{18}F]Fluorocholine PET/CT imaging for the detection of recurrent prostate cancer at PSA relapse: experience in 100 consecutive patients. Eur J Nucl Med Mol Imaging 2006; 33(12):1387–98.

97. Reske SN, Blumstein NM, Neumaier B, et al. Imaging prostate cancer with ^{11}C-choline PET/CT. J Nucl Med 2006;47(8):1249–54.

98. Beheshti M, Vali R, Waldenberger P, et al. The use of F-18 choline PET in the assessment of bone metastases in prostate cancer: correlation with morphological changes on CT. Mol Imaging Biol 2009;11(6):446–54.

99. Tuncel M, Souvatzoglou M, Herrmann K, et al. [^{11}C]Choline positron emission tomography/computed tomography for staging and restaging of patients with advanced prostate cancer. Nucl Med Biol 2008;35(6):689–95.

100. Beheshti M, Vali R, Waldenberger P, et al. Detection of bone metastases in patients with prostate cancer by ^{18}F fluorocholine and ^{18}F fluoride PET-CT: a comparative study. Eur J Nucl Med Mol Imaging 2008;35(10):1766–74.

101. Eschmann SM, Pfannenberg AC, Rieger A, et al. Comparison of [18]C-choline-PET/CT and whole body-MRI for staging of prostate cancer. Nuklearmedizin 2007;46:161–8.

102. Luboldt W, Küfer R, Blumstein N, et al. Prostate carcinoma: diffusion-weighted imaging as potential alternative to conventional MR and [18]C-choline PET/CT for detection of bone metastases. Radiology 2008;249(3):1017–25.

Applications of PET and PET/CT in the Evaluation of Infection and Inflammation in the Skeletal System

Gang Cheng, MD, PhD[a], Pacôme Fosse, MD[b],
Hongming Zhuang, MD, PhD[a], Roland Hustinx, MD, PhD[b],*

KEYWORDS
- Chronic osteomyelitis • PET/CT • Skeletal infection
- Inflammation

Unlike anatomic imaging modalities, which mainly detect structural changes, PET is a molecular imaging technique able to detect the disease in an early stage and long before anatomic changes are visible. It is well known that fluorodeoxyglucose (FDG) accumulates at the sites of various inflammatory and infectious processes.[1,2] FDG-PET or FDG-PET/computed tomography (CT) has been successfully used in the evaluation of various nonosseous soft tissue infections.[3–11] Its application in the evaluation of osseous infection is also promising. This review discusses the potential roles of PET or PET/CT in the evaluation of infection and inflammation in the skeletal system.

CHRONIC OSTEOMYELITIS

The role of PET or PET/CT in the diagnosis of uncomplicated cases of acute osteomyelitis is limited because acute osteomyelitis can be readily diagnosed by routine methods with reasonable accuracy. In contrast, the diagnosis of chronic osteomyelitis is frequently difficult with noninvasive techniques, and the current gold standard of diagnosis is still to obtain a biopsy specimen for

pathologic and microbiological confirmation of the suspected infected bone.[12] Current conventional imaging techniques are unsatisfactory in confirming or excluding chronic osteomyelitis. Although magnetic resonance (MR) imaging and CT can provide outstanding anatomic details, their values in the evaluation of osseous structures that have been changed by previous trauma or surgery are limited, especially in the presence of metallic implants.[13–16] Nuclear medicine imaging has long been used to evaluate chronic osteomyelitis. Three-phase bone scan is an excellent modality with high sensitivity in the evaluation of acute osteomyelitis. However, the specificity of bone scan is not optimal.[17] In addition, the findings of bone scintigraphy were not suitable to monitor the efficacy of the therapy because abnormally increased methylene diphosphonate (MDP) activity can persist for a long period even after successful therapy.[18] Furthermore, traumatized bones following fractures or surgical intervention generally have an extended period of bone remodeling, which causes increased MDP activity[19] and results in difficulty in the evaluation of posttraumatic osteomyelitis. Time-consuming modalities, such as

[a] Department of Radiology, Children's Hospital of Philadelphia, 34th and Civic Center Boulevard, Philadelphia, PA 19104, USA
[b] Division of Nuclear Medicine, University Hospital of Liège, Sart Tilman B35, Liège 4000, Belgium
* Corresponding author. Service de Médecine nucléaire, Centre Hospitalier Universitaire de Liège, Sart Tilman B35, 4000 Liège, Belgique.
E-mail address: rhustinx@chu.ulg.ac.be

PET Clin 5 (2010) 375–385
doi:10.1016/j.cpet.2010.05.003
1556-8598/10/$ – see front matter © 2010 Elsevier Inc. All rights reserved.

Ga 67 scintigraphy[20] or In 111–labeled leukocyte imaging[21] are frequently necessary to supplement bone scan for more accurate diagnosis. Therefore, a more accurate and faster imaging modality is desired.

FDG-PET or FDG-PET/CT has shown to be outstanding in the evaluation of chronic osteomyelitis (**Fig. 1**). Guhlmann and colleagues[22] are the first to test the possibility of using FDG-PET to evaluate osteomyelitis. In their study of 32 patients, they found that FDG-PET had an accuracy of 97% and its sensitivity and specificity were 100% and 92%, respectively. Subsequent investigation confirmed that the accuracy of FDG-PET in the detection of osteomyelitis is high, ranging from 90.9% to 100%.[23–26] Cases of chronic osteomyelitis, which were correctly detected by PET but negative on MRI, had been reported previously.[27] About 3% of skeletal infections occur in the spine, and accurate and early diagnosis of infection in this location remains frequently difficult.[28] Based on the data analyzed from 57 consecutive patients with a history of

previous spinal surgery suspected of spinal infection, de Winter and colleagues[29] reported that sensitivity, specificity, and accuracy of FDG-PET in the evaluation of infection of the spine were 100%, 81%, and 86%, respectively. Other investigators also reported similar results. For example, Schmitz and colleagues[30] showed a sensitivity of 100%, a specificity of 75%, and an accuracy of 94%.

The high accuracy of FDG-PET in the evaluation of osteomyelitis may be attributed to the high resolution of the tomographic nature of the scans in addition to other important factors. One of these factors is that although metal can result in high FDG count due to attenuation, the interpretation of the metabolic images are not affected by metal implants used for fixing fractures (**Fig. 2**),[24,31,32] which makes PET scan an ideal imaging modality to image posttraumatic osteomyelitis. Another factor is the transient nature of increased FDG activity at the fracture site.

It is well known that bone scans remain positive for an extended period of time following

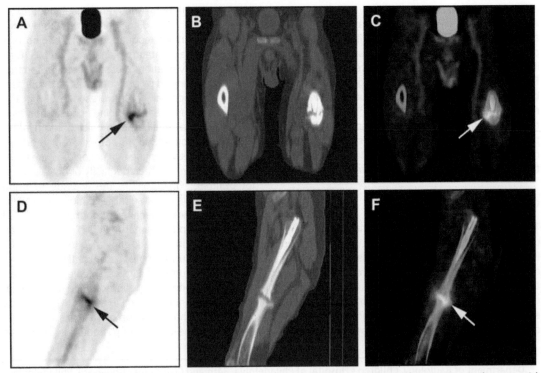

Fig. 1. A 56-year-old man with a history of left femoral fracture status postinternal fixation 8 months ago, with local pain. Radiograph indicated nonunion of fracture. PET/CT scan was performed to evaluate possible infection. (*A*) Coronal PET image. (*B*) Coronal low-dose CT image (bone window). (*C*) Fused coronal PET/CT image. (*D*) Sagittal PET image. (*E*) Sagittal low-dose CT image (bone window). (*F*) Fused sagittal PET/CT image. The PET images show focally increased FDG uptake in the fracture site of the mid–left femur (*arrows*), whereas CT images indicated fracture nonunion (*B, E*). The findings were compatible with osteomyelitis at the fracture site, which was later confirmed at surgery.

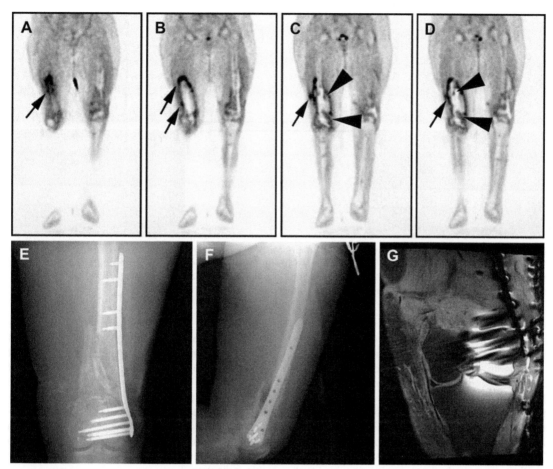

Fig. 2. A 50-year-old woman with a history of a gunshot to both lower extremities and bilateral comminuted femoral fractures extending to the bilateral femoral condyles 1 month ago, status postbilateral open reduction/internal fixations, with clinical suspicion of osteomyelitis. (*A–D*) Selected coronal images of FDG-PET from the anterior to the posterior. Abnormally increased FDG uptake is visualized in the soft tissues surrounding the mid/distal right femur (*arrows*). In addition, some of the tracer activity tracks inside the bony structure (*arrowheads*) indicate osteomyelitis with surrounding soft tissue infection. Milder FDG activity is seen surrounding the left femur and the left knee, consistent with inflammation caused by fractures and internal fixation. (*E, F*) Anterior/posterior and lateral radiographic views of the right distal femur, showing the fracture and fixation. (*G*) MR image performed on the same day, which is nondiagnostic and limited by extensive metallic artifact arising from orthopedic fixation devices. Surgical biopsy was performed 4 days later, and osseous infection with *Klebsiella pneumoniae* and *Enterococcus* spp was confirmed.

fractures.[19] However, FDG-PET is positive at the fracture site for only a relatively short period (**Fig. 3**). In 1989, Paul and colleagues[33] were the first to notice that there was no increased FDG activity at the site of the healing fracture. However, in 1994, Meyer and colleagues[34] found significantly increased FDG in a 2-week-old fracture of the clavicle and scapula in a 24-year-old man. The first convincing investigation was conducted by Schmitz and colleagues.[35] In their study, 17 patients with compression fractures of the vertebral bodies were evaluated by bone scintigraphy and FDG-PET scan. MDP bone scans showed positive results in all 17 patients. In contrast, PET scans showed positive results in 5 and negative results in 12. All 12 patients had uncomplicated compression fractures. Of the 5 patients with positive PET scans, 3 had spondylodiscitis and 1 had pathologic fracture. Zhuang and colleagues[36] analyzed FDG uptake levels in the fracture sites of 37 patients and compared those with the time interval between the fracture and PET scan. Among these patients, 14 had fractures within 3 months before FDG-PET and 23 had fractures more than 3 months before FDG-PET. FDG-PET showed no abnormally increased uptake at the known fracture or surgical sites in 30 of these patients. In the 23 patients with fractures more than 3 months

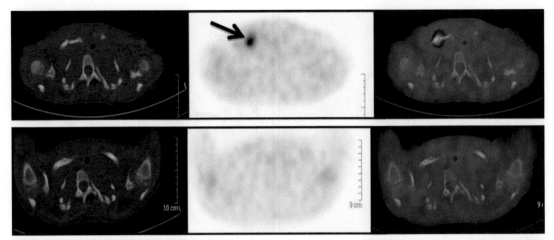

Fig. 3. (*Top panel*) The bone window of the CT images (*left*) showed clear right clavicle fracture, which occurred 10 days before the PET/CT scan. On PET (*middle*) and fusion (*right*) images, there was intense FDG activity at the fracture site (*arrow*). (*Bottom panel*) On follow-up PET study, which was acquired 7 weeks after the first PET/CT scan, the abnormal FDG activity was no longer visualized at the fracture site.

old, all but 1 showed normal uptake. Furthermore, the positive FDG uptake in this exception was a result of complicating osteomyelitis. In the 14 patients with a history of fracture less than 3 months old, only 6 had abnormally increased FDG uptake. The authors concluded that following fractures, FDG uptake is expected to be normal within 3 months unless the process is complicated by infection or malignancy.[36] The results of these retrospective clinical investigations were further confirmed by well-controlled animal experiments.[37] Koort and colleagues[37] compared FDG uptake pattern in 8 rabbits with normal fracture healing and 8 rabbits with osteomyelitis. They found that uncomplicated bone healing was associated with a temporary increase in FDG uptake at 3 weeks, but levels returned almost to normal by 6 weeks. In contrast, osteomyelitis resulted in an intense continuous uptake of FDG, which was higher than that of healing and intact bones at 3 and 6 weeks ($P<.001$).

Because the fracture-related FDG activity is transient and increased FDG activity caused by metal attenuation does not affect PET interpretation, FDG-PET is particularly useful in the evaluation of posttraumatic osteomyelitis. In an investigation involving 33 patients with trauma suspected of having chronic osteomyelitis, Hartmann and colleagues[31] found that sensitivity, specificity, and accuracy for FDG-PET/CT were 94%, 87%, and 91%, respectively. FDG-PET may also correctly identify chronic posttraumatic osteomyelitis in patients with negative MR imaging findings and antigranulocyte antibody scintigraphy.[27] Experimental studies in rodents

suggest that Ga 68 PET might be helpful for evaluating possible osteomyelitis at the site of a very recent fracture. Healing bones without infection showed slightly elevated uptake of FDG but not Ga 68, whereas FDG and Ga 68 had intense activity at the sites of osteomyelitis.[38] It is perceived that FDG imaging is superior to labeled leukocyte scintigraphy in the diagnosis of chronic osteomyelitis and therefore should be considered the method of choice for this indication.[26]

Although most studies regarding the FDG activity in osteomyelitis were performed using only a PET scanner, it is certain that the CT portion of the PET/CT can further increase the accuracy of the scan. For example, it is known that nonossifying fibroma can result in elevated FDG activity,[39–41] but the characteristic pattern of nonossifying fibroma on CT helps PET/CT readers exclude other osseous pathologies, including osteomyelitis (**Fig. 4**).

Because malignant and infectious processes may result in increased FDG activity, occasionally malignant lesions in the bone are misinterpreted as osteomyelitis.[42] Some investigators have found that dual-phase FDG-PET imaging has the potential to distinguish osteomyelitis from malignant osseous lesions because FDG uptake levels remained stable or decreased in the later time compared with the early time imaging in osteomyelitis but increased significantly in malignant lesions.[43]

DIABETIC FOOT

Diabetic foot is a complicated joint and bone disorder in the foot in patients with diabetes. Up to 10% of the patients with diabetes will develop

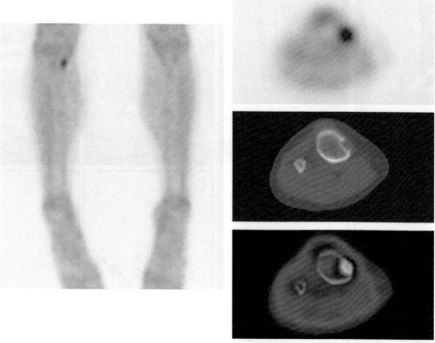

Fig. 4. Projection (*left*) and transaxial PET (*top right*) image revealed an abnormal activity in the proximal right tibia, suspected of osteomyelitis. However, on CT image (*center right*), the lesion is eccentric with central radiolucency and cortical defect, which is typical for nonossifying fibroma. Because on fusion image (*bottom right*) the FDG activity corresponded well to the nonossifying fibroma, a false-positive interpretation of osteomyelitis was avoided.

foot ulcers, and approximately 15% of these patients will develop osteomyelitis.[44] Osteomyelitis in such patients is frequently nonresponsive to antibiotic therapy and eventually mandates surgical intervention. Early diagnosis of osteomyelitis in patients with diabetic foot is crucial because intense but expensive antibiotic therapy early can be curative and prevents amputation, which is the most feared complication in these patients. Therefore, the importance of accurate early diagnosis of osteomyelitis in this patient population cannot be overestimated. Some investigators suggest that FDG-PET might be able to play important roles in the evaluation of diabetic foot.

FDG-PET was reported to be able to reliably differentiate between osteomyelitis and infection of the surrounding soft tissue (**Fig. 5**).[45] FDG-PET has the potential to differentiate uncomplicated Charcot neuroarthropathy from osteomyelitis and soft tissue infection[46] or septic arthritis.[47] Keidar and colleagues[48] studied 18 clinically suspected sites of infection using PET/CT for suspected osteomyelitis complicating diabetic foot disease. PET detected 14 foci of increased FDG uptake consistent with infection. PET/CT correctly localized 8 foci to bone, indicating osteomyelitis. PET/CT correctly excluded osteomyelitis in 5 foci, with

the abnormal FDG uptake limited to infected soft tissues only. One site of mildly increased focal FDG uptake was localized by PET/CT to diabetic osteoarthropathy changes demonstrated on CT. Four patients showed no abnormally increased FDG uptake and no further evidence of an infectious process on clinical and imaging follow-up. The authors concluded that FDG-PET/CT enables accurate differentiation between osteomyelitis and soft tissue infection in patients with diabetic foot.[48]

In a prospective investigation, Hopfner and colleagues[49] compared FDG-PET and MR imaging in the diagnosis of Charcot neuropathy of the foot requiring operative treatment. Of 39 Charcot lesions confirmed at surgery, 37 were detected by FDG-PET and 31 by MR imaging. The differentiation between Charcot neuroarthropathy and florid osteomyelitis provides the surgeon with important additional information that often is unavailable from MR imaging. Because it provides important additional data, the authors think that PET may be preferable to radiography and MR imaging in the preoperative evaluation of patients.[49]

The largest investigation so far is by Nawaz and colleagues.[50] In this prospective study, 110 consecutive patients with diabetic foot were

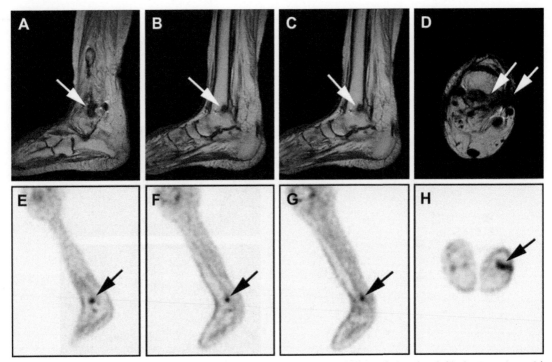

Fig. 5. A 75-year-old woman with antecedents of diabetes and resection of the distal fibula, presents with a chronic wound in the left ankle with clinical suspicion of osteomyelitis of the left foot. MR imaging (*A–D*) and FDG-PET (*E–H*) images are shown. MR imaging demonstrated decreased T1-weighted signal intensity extending from the lateral skin margin to the lateral portion of the tibia/tibiotalar joint (*white arrows*), consistent with a chronic sinus tract without evidence of osteomyelitis or abscess. However, FDG-PET scan performed within 2 weeks of MR imaging demonstrated linearly increased radiotracer uptake in the soft tissues of the left fibular malleolus extending to the distal tibia/tibiotalar joint (*black arrows*), consistent with an active soft tissue infection and possibly osteomyelitis. (*A–C*) Selected sagittal sections of MR image, from lateral to medial of the left ankle. (*D*) Transaxial section of MR image. (*E–G*) Selected sagittal sections of FDG-PET from lateral to medial of the left ankle. (*H*) Transaxial section of FDG-PET. Surgical debridement was performed subsequently, which showed acute soft tissue infection with adjacent osteomyelits and formation of granulomatous tissues. Microbiological culture from bone specimen was positive for *Staphylococcus aureus*.

enrolled. FDG-PET and MR imaging were performed in each patient to evaluate possible osteomyelitis. The results showed that FDG-PET correctly diagnosed osteomyelitis in 21 of 26 patients and correctly excluded it in 74 of 80, with sensitivity, specificity, positive predictive value (PPV), negative predictive value (NPV), and accuracy of 81%, 93%, 78%, 94%, and 90%, respectively. MR imaging correctly diagnosed osteomyelitis in 20 of 22 patients and correctly excluded it in 56 of 72, with sensitivity, specificity, PPV, NPV, and accuracy of 91%, 78%, 56%, 97%, and 81%, respectively.

ARTHROPLASTY-ASSOCIATED INFECTION

Successful joint replacement has improved the quality of life for many patients with degenerative arthritis. However, a small proportion of the patients suffer long-standing postsurgical pain. Pain is mostly caused by biomechanical failure of the prostheses or loosening or occasionally by periprosthetic infection. Clinically, loosening and periprosthetic infection present similar symptoms, and it is a major diagnostic challenge to distinguish these 2 different clinical entities.

Zhuang and colleagues[51] were among those who first tried to use FDG-PET to evaluate arthroplasty-associated infection in a large patient population. In their investigation, 62 patients with 74 prostheses (36 knee and 38 hip prostheses) were included. FDG-PET showed an overall sensitivity of 90.5% and specificity of 81.8%. Reinartz and colleagues[52] studied 92 possibly infected hip prostheses with FDG-PET scan and reported sensitivity, specificity, and accuracy of 93.9%, 94.9%, and 94.6%, respectively. Nonspecific FDG uptake after hip arthroplasty can last for as long as 2 decades in patients without any symptoms.[53] This nonspecific FDG activity is generally located in the regions adjacent to the head and neck of the hip prosthesis and should not be interpreted as a sign of infection (**Fig. 6**). The elevated FDG activity caused by periprosthetic infection should be in the periprosthetic soft tissue (**Fig. 7**) or arthroplasty interface.[52,54–56]

The experience of using FDG-PET in the evaluation of knee prostheses is much more limited than that in hip prostheses. The reported overall accuracy of FDG-PET in the evaluation of knee prostheses is also lower than for hip prostheses,[51,57] which is likely because of the lack of an optimal diagnostic standard. However, there are some promising reports. For example, Manthey and colleagues[58] evaluated 14 painful knee arthroplasties and found both sensitivity and specificity of 100%. However, further investigation is necessary to establish or disprove the utility of FDG-PET in the evaluation of painful knee prostheses.

RHEUMATOID ARTHRITIS

Rheumatoid arthritis (RA) is the most prevalent inflammatory joint disease and affects 1% of the population. It is an autoimmune systemic disease characterized by chronic inflammation of the synovium, with a massive leukocyte infiltration, neovascularization, and proliferation of the synovial membrane. The natural evolution of the disease leads to the erosion of the cartilage and bone, resulting in severe disability. The management of RA has greatly evolved with the advent of the biologic therapies, in particular tumor necrosis factor (TNF) α inhibitors. These treatments may prevent joint destruction and significantly improve the quality of life and functional performances of patients with RA. Disease activity is primarily assessed using a composite scale, the Disease Activity

Scale (DAS) 28, which integrates clinical and biologic parameters of inflammation. Ultrasonography (US) and MR imaging are imaging methods capable of indirectly identifying inflammatory processes using synovial thickness measurements and power Doppler signal for US[59] and semiautomated methods for characterizing dynamic contrast enhancement for MR imaging.[60] However, both methods have limitations because US is highly operator dependent and MR imaging usually explores a limited number of joints.

Palmer and colleagues[61] first described the feasibility of using FDG-PET for quantifying inflammation in wrist joints in patients with rheumatoid or psoriatic arthritis. Metabolic measurements were closely correlated with the volume of enhancing pannus measured by MR imaging, and imaging parameters were also associated with clinical signs of inflammation, such as pain, tenderness, and swelling. Similar results were obtained in the knees of 16 patients with active RA who were prospectively investigated by physical examination, PET, US, and MR imaging.[62] Standardized uptake values (SUVs) were significantly correlated to MR imaging parameters, synovial thickness, and serum levels of C-reactive protein (CRP) and matrix metalloproteinase-3, a synovium-derived parameter reflecting joint inflammation. Overall, the observations suggest strong relationships between the depth of the synovitis measured by US, its metabolic activity measured by PET, and its vascularization and leukocyte infiltration reflected by the dynamic MR imaging parameters. PET, especially newer devices, is capable of exploring multiple joints in a reasonable amount of time. This capability was shown in 21 patients

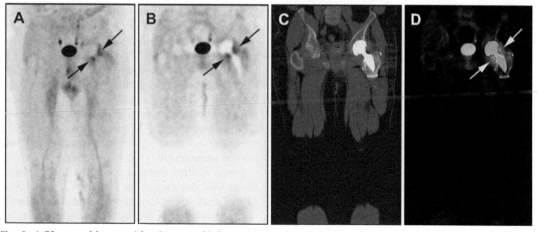

Fig. 6. A 50-year-old man with a history of left total hip arthroplasty 3 years ago. (*A*) Maximum intensity projection FDG-PET image. (*B*) Coronal FDG-PET image. (*C*) Coronal low-dose CT image (bone window). (*D*) Fused PET/CT image. PET images demonstrate focally increased FDG uptake near the neck of the prosthesis (*arrows*), indicating reactive changes to prosthesis rather than infection.

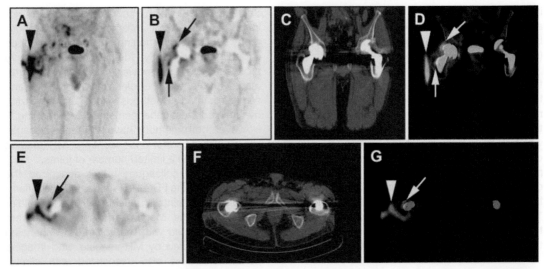

Fig. 7. A 55-year-old patient with a history of bilateral total hip replacement, with right side pain. PET/CT was performed to evaluate possible infection. (*A*) Maximum intensity projection PET image. (*B*) Coronal PET image. (*C*) Coronal low-dose CT image (bone window). (*D*) Fused coronal PET/CT image. (*E*) Transaxial PET image. (*F*) Transaxial low-dose CT image (bone window). (*G*) Fused transaxial PET/CT image. This study shows intense and heterogeneous tracer uptake in the soft tissues involving the skin and extending to the right hip (*arrowheads*). Activity in the bone/prosthetic interface is also noted (*arrows*). These findings are consistent with periprosthetic infection. Surgery was performed 6 days later with debridement and replacement of prostheses. Pathologic examination was consistent with acute infection, and culture confirmed infection with *Staphylococcus aureus*.

with RA studied using clinical joint examination, US, and PET.[63] Knees were evaluated in all patients in addition to either wrists and hands metacarpophalangeal and proximal interphalangeal joints or ankles and the first metatarsophalangeal joints according to clinical complaints. Again, PET positivity was closely correlated to increased synovial thickness on US and to physical examination, that is, presence of tenderness or swelling. Furthermore, a global RA PET activity index obtained by calculating the number of PET-positive joints per patient and the cumulative SUV in these joints was highly correlated with the number of tender and swollen joints, patient's and physician's global assessment scores, biologic parameters of inflammation (erythrocyte sedimentation rate and CRP levels), US parameters (number of US-positive joints and the cumulative synovial thickness), and the composite indices of RA disease activity such as the DAS28. PET seems suitable for quantifying the disease activity in multiple joints in patients with RA. Although FDG uptake is increased in most inflamed joints, such observation is obviously not specific to RA. A similar level of uptake was found in joints of patients with active, subclinical osteoarthritis.[64]

At this stage, PET essentially remains an experimental method in patients with RA. The most likely clinical indication to emerge is the evaluation of the

response to treatment. The development of effective but costly biologic treatments for RA has prompted the interest of new methods for assessing their efficacy in addition to the crude clinical counts of tender and swollen joints and to the late radiologic measures of erosions. Goerres and colleagues[65] evaluated 7 patients with RA before and after 12 weeks of treatment with infliximab. Metabolic changes correlated with clinical assessment in 78% of joints. The reduction of FDG uptake was noted not only in joints but also in bursae of 3 responders and in tendon sheaths of 4 responders. This limited series confirms the potential of PET for a whole-body assessment of RA disease activity at baseline and after anti-TNF treatment. At this point, however, the clinical relevance of PET is not established, that is, whether the metabolic assessment of RA disease activity can distinguish anti-TNF responders and nonresponders earlier or in a more sensitive way than clinical assessment.

These studies were all performed using standalone PET devices. In all likelihood, the addition of the anatomic information provided by the CT study should further enhance the diagnostic accuracy and interobserver reproducibility. Initial results are encouraging, but remain limited (**Fig. 8**).[66] Other possible developments may stem from alternative tracers. Roivanen and

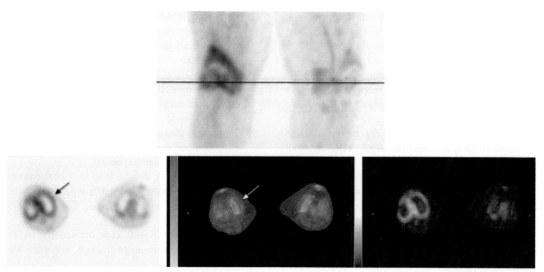

Fig. 8. Active synovitis in a patient with RA refractory to anti–TNF-α treatment. The 3-dimensional projection image (*top*) depicts a typical pattern of synovitis of the right knee. Corresponding transaxial slices of the PET, CT, and fused PET/CT images (*bottom panel*) show that the increased FDG levels correspond to thickened synovium (*arrows*).

colleagues[67] showed a strong correlation between FDG uptake, ^{11}C-choline uptake, and synovial volume measured by MR imaging in a series of 10 patients. More recently, specific targeting of macrophages with (R)-[^{11}C]PK11195, has been proposed. This ligand binds to the peripheral benzodiazepine receptor, which is mainly expressed by macrophages and monocytes and is thus considered as a marker for inflammation. Preliminary results are highly encouraging, although further validation remains needed.[68,69]

REFERENCES

1. Zhuang H, Alavi A. 18-Fluorodeoxyglucose positron emission tomographic imaging in the detection and monitoring of infection and inflammation. Semin Nucl Med 2002;32:47–59.

2. Kumar R, Basu S, Torigian D, et al. Role of modern imaging techniques for diagnosis of infection in the era of 18F-fluorodeoxyglucose positron emission tomography. Clin Microbiol Rev 2008;21:209–24.

3. Scharko AM, Perlman SB, Pyzalski RW, et al. Whole-body positron emission tomography in patients with HIV-1 infection. Lancet 2003;362:959–61.

4. Simons KS, Pickkers P, Bleeker-Rovers CP, et al. F-18-fluorodeoxyglucose positron emission tomography combined with CT in critically ill patients with suspected infection. Intensive Care Med 2010;36:504–11.

5. Klein M, Cohen-Cymberknoh M, Armoni S, et al. 18F-fluorodeoxyglucose-PET/CT imaging of lungs in patients with cystic fibrosis. Chest 2009;136:1220–8.

6. Wan DQ, Joseph UA, Barron BJ, et al. Ventriculoperitoneal shunt catheter and cerebral spinal fluid infection initially detected by FDG PET/CT scan. Clin Nucl Med 2009;34:464–5.

7. Spacek M, Belohlavek O, Votrubova J, et al. Diagnostics of "non-acute" vascular prosthesis infection using 18F-FDG PET/CT: our experience with 96 prostheses. Eur J Nucl Med Mol Imaging 2009;36:850–8.

8. Choi SJ, Lee JS, Cheong MH, et al. F-18 FDG PET/CT in the management of infected abdominal aortic aneurysm due to Salmonella. Clin Nucl Med 2008;33:492–5.

9. Park CH, Lee MH, Oh CG. F-18 FDG positron emission tomographic imaging in bilateral iliopsoas abscesses. Clin Nucl Med 2002;27:680–1.

10. Sheehy N, Israel DA. Acute varicella infection mimics recurrent Hodgkin's disease on F-18 FDG PET/CT. Clin Nucl Med 2007;32:820–1.

11. Louis E, Ancion G, Colard A, et al. Noninvasive assessment of Crohn's disease intestinal lesions with (18)F-FDG PET/CT. J Nucl Med 2007;48:1053–9.

12. Fluckiger U, Zimmerli W. Diagnosis and follow-up management of postoperative bacterial osteitis. Orthopade 2004;33:416–23.

13. Crim JR, Seeger LL. Imaging evaluation of osteomyelitis. Crit Rev Diagn Imaging 1994;35:201–56.

14. Erdman WA, Tamburro F, Jayson HT, et al. Osteomyelitis: characteristics and pitfalls of diagnosis with MR imaging. Radiology 1991;180:533–9.

15. Kaim A, Ledermann HP, Bongartz G, et al. Chronic post-traumatic osteomyelitis of the lower extremity: comparison of magnetic resonance

imaging and combined bone scintigraphy/immunoscintigraphy with radiolabelled monoclonal antigranulocyte antibodies. Skeletal Radiol 2000;29: 378–86.

16. Ledermann HP, Kaim A, Bongartz G, et al. Pitfalls and limitations of magnetic resonance imaging in chronic posttraumatic osteomyelitis. Eur Radiol 2000;10:1815–23.

17. Schauwecker DS, Braunstein EM, Wheat LJ. Diagnostic imaging of osteomyelitis. Infect Dis Clin North Am 1990;4:441–63.

18. Schauwecker DS. The scintigraphic diagnosis of osteomyelitis. AJR Am J Roentgenol 1992;158:9–18.

19. Matin P. The appearance of bone scans following fractures, including immediate and long-term studies. J Nucl Med 1979;20:1227–31.

20. Hartshorne MF, Graham G, Lancaster J, et al. Gallium-67/technetium-99m methylene diphosphonate ratio imaging: early rabbit osteomyelitis and fracture. J Nucl Med 1985;26:272–7.

21. Datz FL. Indium-111-labeled leukocytes for the detection of infection: current status. Semin Nucl Med 1994;24:92–109.

22. Guhlmann A, Brecht-Krauss D, Suger G, et al. Chronic osteomyelitis: detection with FDG PET and correlation with histopathologic findings. Radiology 1998;206:749–54.

23. Zhuang H, Duarte PS, Pourdehand M, et al. Exclusion of chronic osteomyelitis with F-18 fluorodeoxyglucose positron emission tomographic imaging. Clin Nucl Med 2000;25:281–4.

24. Kalicke T, Schmitz A, Risse JH, et al. Fluorine-18 fluorodeoxyglucose PET in infectious bone diseases: results of histologically confirmed cases. Eur J Nucl Med 2000;27:524–8.

25. de Winter F, Van de Wiele C, Vandenberghe S, et al. Coincidence camera FDG imaging for the diagnosis of chronic orthopedic infections: a feasibility study. J Comput Assist Tomogr 2001;25:184–9.

26. Meller J, Koster G, Liersch T, et al. Chronic bacterial osteomyelitis: prospective comparison of (18)F-FDG imaging with a dual-head coincidence camera and (111)In-labelled autologous leucocyte scintigraphy. Eur J Nucl Med Mol Imaging 2002; 29:53–60.

27. Robiller FC, Stumpe KD, Kossmann T, et al. Chronic osteomyelitis of the femur: value of PET imaging. Eur Radiol 2000;10:855–8.

28. Arizono T, Oga M, Shiota E, et al. Differentiation of vertebral osteomyelitis and tuberculous spondylitis by magnetic resonance imaging. Int Orthop 1995; 19:319–22.

29. De Winter F, Gemmel F, Van De Wiele C, et al. 18-Fluorine fluorodeoxyglucose positron emission tomography for the diagnosis of infection in the postoperative spine. Spine (Phila Pa 1976) 2003;28: 1314–9.

30. Schmitz A, Risse JH, Grunwald F, et al. Fluorine-18 fluorodeoxyglucose positron emission tomography findings in spondylodiscitis: preliminary results. Eur Spine J 2001;10:534–9.

31. Hartmann A, Eid K, Dora C, et al. Diagnostic value of 18F-FDG PET/CT in trauma patients with suspected chronic osteomyelitis. Eur J Nucl Med Mol Imaging 2007;34:704–14.

32. Trampuz A, Zimmerli W. Diagnosis and treatment of infections associated with fracture-fixation devices. Injury 2006;37(Suppl 2):S59–66.

33. Paul R, Ahonen A, Virtama P, et al. F-18 fluorodeoxyglucose: its potential in differentiating between stress fracture and neoplasia. Clin Nucl Med 1989;14:906–8.

34. Meyer M, Gast T, Raja S, et al. Increased F-18 FDG accumulation in an acute fracture. Clin Nucl Med 1994;19:13–4.

35. Schmitz A, Risse JH, Textor J, et al. FDG-PET findings of vertebral compression fractures in osteoporosis: preliminary results. Osteoporos Int 2002;13: 755–61.

36. Zhuang H, Sam JW, Chacko TK, et al. Rapid normalization of osseous FDG uptake following traumatic or surgical fractures. Eur J Nucl Med Mol Imaging 2003;30:1096–103.

37. Koort JK, Makinen TJ, Knuuti J, et al. Comparative 18F-FDG PET of experimental Staphylococcus aureus osteomyelitis and normal bone healing. J Nucl Med 2004;45:1406–11.

38. Makinen TJ, Lankinen P, Poyhonen T, et al. Comparison of 18F-FDG and 68Ga PET imaging in the assessment of experimental osteomyelitis due to Staphylococcus aureus. Eur J Nucl Med Mol Imaging 2005;32:1259–68.

39. Goodin GS, Shulkin BL, Kaufman RA, et al. PET/CT characterization of fibroosseous defects in children: 18F-FDG uptake can mimic metastatic disease. AJR Am J Roentgenol 2006;187:1124–8.

40. von Falck C, Rosenthal H, Gratz KF, et al. Nonossifying fibroma can mimic residual lymphoma in FDG PET: additional value of combined PET/CT. Clin Nucl Med 2007;32:640–2.

41. Iagaru A, Henderson R. PET/CT follow-up in nonossifying fibroma. AJR Am J Roentgenol 2006; 187:830–2.

42. Chamroonrat W, Houseni M, Bing Z, et al. Non-Hodgkin's lymphoma of the bone can mimic osteomyelitis on FDG PET. Clin Nucl Med 2007;32:252–4.

43. Sahlmann CO, Siefker U, Lehmann K, et al. Dual time point 2-[18F]fluoro-2'-deoxyglucose positron emission tomography in chronic bacterial osteomyelitis. Nucl Med Commun 2004;25:819–23.

44. Boulton AJ, Vileikyte L. The diabetic foot: the scope of the problem. J Fam Pract 2000;49:S3–8.

45. Guhlmann A, Brecht-Krauss D, Suger G, et al. Fluorine-18-FDG PET and technetium-99m

antigranulocyte antibody scintigraphy in chronic osteomyelitis. J Nucl Med 1998;39:2145–52.

46. Basu S, Chryssikos T, Houseni M, et al. Potential role of FDG PET in the setting of diabetic neuro-osteoarthropathy: can it differentiate uncomplicated Charcot's neuroarthropathy from osteomyelitis and soft-tissue infection? Nucl Med Commun 2007;28: 465–72.

47. Alnafisi N, Yun M, Alavi A. F-18 FDG positron emission tomography to differentiate diabetic osteoarthropathy from septic arthritis. Clin Nucl Med 2001;26: 638–9.

48. Keidar Z, Militianu D, Melamed E, et al. The diabetic foot: initial experience with 18F-FDG PET/CT. J Nucl Med 2005;46:444–9.

49. Hopfner S, Krolak C, Kessler S, et al. Preoperative imaging of Charcot neuroarthropathy in diabetic patients: comparison of ring PET, hybrid PET, and magnetic resonance imaging. Foot Ankle Int 2004; 25:890–5.

50. Nawaz A, Torigian DA, Siegelman ES, et al. Diagnostic performance of FDG-PET, MRI, and plain film radiography (PFR) for the diagnosis of osteomyelitis in the diabetic foot. Mol Imaging Biol 2010;12: 335–42.

51. Zhuang H, Duarte PS, Pourdehnad M, et al. The promising role of 18F-FDG PET in detecting infected lower limb prosthesis implants. J Nucl Med 2001;42:44–8.

52. Reinartz P, Mumme T, Hermanns B, et al. Radionuclide imaging of the painful hip arthroplasty: positron-emission tomography versus triple-phase bone scanning. J Bone Joint Surg Br 2005;87:465–70.

53. Zhuang H, Chacko TK, Hickeson M, et al. Persistent non-specific FDG uptake on PET imaging following hip arthroplasty. Eur J Nucl Med Mol Imaging 2002;29:1328–33.

54. Mumme T, Reinartz P, Alfer J, et al. Diagnostic values of positron emission tomography versus triple-phase bone scan in hip arthroplasty loosening. Arch Orthop Trauma Surg 2005;125:322–9.

55. Chacko TK, Zhuang H, Stevenson K, et al. The importance of the location of fluorodeoxyglucose uptake in periprosthetic infection in painful hip prostheses. Nucl Med Commun 2002;23:851–5.

56. Chacko TK, Zhuang H, Nakhoda KZ, et al. Applications of fluorodeoxyglucose positron emission tomography in the diagnosis of infection. Nucl Med Commun 2003;24:615–24.

57. Stumpe KD, Romero J, Ziegler O, et al. The value of FDG-PET in patients with painful total knee arthroplasty. Eur J Nucl Med Mol Imaging 2006;33:1218–25.

58. Manthey N, Reinhard P, Moog F, et al. The use of [18 F]fluorodeoxyglucose positron emission tomography to differentiate between synovitis, loosening and infection of hip and knee prostheses. Nucl Med Commun 2002;23:645–53.

59. Ribbens C, André B, Marcelis S, et al. Rheumatoid hand joint synovitis: gray-scale and power Doppler US quantifications following anti-tumor necrosis factor-alpha treatment: pilot study. Radiology 2003; 229:562–9.

60. Bird P, Lassere M, Shnier R, et al. Computerized measurement of magnetic resonance imaging erosion volumes in patients with rheumatoid arthritis: a comparison with existing magnetic resonance imaging scoring systems and standard clinical outcome measures. Arthritis Rheum 2003;48: 614–24.

61. Palmer WE, Rosenthal DI, Schoenberg OI, et al. Quantification of inflammation in the wrist with gadolinium-enhanced MR imaging and PET with 2-[F-18]-fluoro-2-deoxy-D-glucose. Radiology 1995; 196:647–55.

62. Beckers C, Jeukens X, Ribbens C, et al. (18)F-FDG PET imaging of rheumatoid knee synovitis correlates with dynamic magnetic resonance and sonographic assessments as well as with the serum level of metalloproteinase-3. Eur J Nucl Med Mol Imaging 2006;33:275–80.

63. Beckers C, Ribbens C, André B, et al. Assessment of disease activity in rheumatoid arthritis with (18)F-FDG PET. J Nucl Med 2004;45:956–64.

64. Elzinga EH, van der Laken CJ, Comans EF, et al. 2-Deoxy-2-[F-18]fluoro-D-glucose joint uptake on positron emission tomography images: rheumatoid arthritis versus osteoarthritis. Mol Imaging Biol 2007;9:357–60.

65. Goerres GW, Forster A, Uebelhart D, et al. F-18 FDG whole-body PET for the assessment of disease activity in patients with rheumatoid arthritis. Clin Nucl Med 2006;31:386–90.

66. Kubota K, Ito K, Morooka M, et al. Whole-body FDG-PET/CT on rheumatoid arthritis of large joints. Ann Nucl Med 2009;23:783–91.

67. Roivainen A, Parkkola R, Yli-Kerttula T, et al. Use of positron emission tomography with methyl-11C-choline and 2-18F-fluoro-2-deoxy-D-glucose in comparison with magnetic resonance imaging for the assessment of inflammatory proliferation of synovium. Arthritis Rheum 2003;48:3077–84.

68. Kropholler MA, Boellaard R, Elzinga EH, et al. Quantification of (R)-[11C] PK11195 binding in rheumatoid arthritis. Eur J Nucl Med Mol Imaging 2009;36: 624–31.

69. van der Laken CJ, Elzinga EH, Kropholler MA, et al. Noninvasive imaging of macrophages in rheumatoid synovitis using 11C-(R)-PK11195 and positron emission tomography. Arthritis Rheum 2008;58:3350–5.

INDEX

Note: Page numbers of article titles are in **boldface** type.

PET Clin 5 (2010) 387–390
doi:10.1016/S1556-8598(10)00084-2

Moving?

Make sure your subscription moves with you!

To notify us of your new address, find your **Clinics Account Number** (located on your mailing label above your name), and contact customer service at:

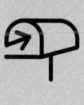

Email: journalscustomerservice-usa@elsevier.com

800-654-2452 (subscribers in the U.S. & Canada)
314-447-8871 (subscribers outside of the U.S. & Canada)

Fax number: 314-447-8029

Elsevier Health Sciences Division
Subscription Customer Service
3251 Riverport Lane
Maryland Heights, MO 63043

*To ensure uninterrupted delivery of your subscription, please notify us at least 4 weeks in advance of move.

ELSEVIER

Printed and bound by CPI Group (UK) Ltd, Croydon, CR0 4YY

03/10/2024

01040356-0012